"Dear Thor, I want to than ▮▮▮▮▮▮ transforming my life comp ▮▮▮ ▮▮▮ ▮▮▮▮▮ ▮▮▮▮▮! book, it took me but a few months to completely change my lifestyle. Now, I am on my seventh month and going super strong. Recently, I began applying the principles of raw food living to my clients. They are soaking it up and the results are amazing. Never in my 15-year career have I seen such transformations. What a difference your book has made in my health and life."

— Alex Poptodorov, Bodybuilder and Personal Trainer

"Raw Power! Protein has been an outstanding addition to my diet over the past couple of years. Not only has Raw Power! been the high quality source of plant-based protein I was looking for, but I have also enjoyed receiving the nutritional benefits from the superfood blend. Raw Power! is a key ingredient I use when making smoothies, energy/protein bars, and it is very good when mixed with water alone. I recommend Raw Power! to other athletes and people who are looking to supplement their diet with a product that promotes nutritional excellence!!!"

— Nick Goings, NFL Running Back, Carolina Panthers

"Thor, your Raw Power! Protein powder has the most amazing ingredients. Thanks for your awesome creation. It rocks! Protein powder doesn't get much better than this! I put it in my smoothie every day following my workout."

— Kathy Feldman Leveque, National Fitness Competitor, Author of The Raw Crunch Diet, and Creator of Raw Crunch Bars

"I love this product," exclaimed Mike Adams, natural health author and raw foods enthusiast. "Thor's Raw Power! Protein is the first raw, vegan, organic protein powder I've ever seen, and it's perfect for those of us who eat right and train hard."

While bodybuilders may not care what they put into their bodies as long as it boosts muscle mass, natural health enthusiasts like Mike Adams are notoriously choosy in deciding what to consume. "I need supplemental protein because I train five days a week and I refuse to eat red meat for a number of reasons, both nutritional and ethical. Finding Thor's Raw Power! was like discovering nutritional treasure. I've made it a regular part of my morning smoothie drinks from the first day I brought it home."

"The taste of Raw Power! Protein took a little while to get used to as it is a very natural product. However, now I really like the protein powder. It mixes well with fruits and it goes down easy and does not have a chemical artificial feel to it as most protein powders do."

— Mike Mahler, Strength Coach

"Have incorporated Thor's Hammer tablets into my daily diet. I'm working overseas and will have to order ahead of time so as to not interrupt my intake. Great stuff. Will be utilizing your services into the ever. Good Health!"

"As a former bodybuilder, olympic weight-lifter, and a present 100% raw-foodist, I think your book Raw Power! is the best I've ever read on the subject—it's great—keep it up!"

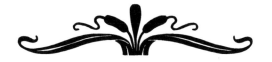

Raw Power!

The Power of Raw Foods, Superfoods and Building Strength and Muscle Naturally

Thor Bazler

Raw Power Publishing
Coeur d'Alene, Idaho

www.rawpower.com

Raw Power!
by Thor Bazler

Disclaimer:
Information contained within this book is provided for informational purposes only and is not intended as a substitute for the advice provided by your physician or other healthcare professional. Information in this book should not be used for diagnosing or treating a health problem or disease, or prescribing any medication or other treatment.

First Edition: August 1, 1998
Fourth Edition: May 1, 2011
ISBN #: 978-0-9815128-0-8

Thor's Raw Power Protein and Superfood products, and many other foods and products mentioned in this book, are now available online.

Please visit our Raw Organic Superstore at:

www.rawpower.com

or call us at 1-877-846-7708

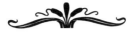

Table of Contents

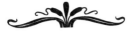

Introduction:

My Health Food Story

Hello Reader, and thank you for taking the time out of your busy life to read this book. As they say, "So many books, so little time." If you are reading this book, you must have an interest in health, diet, fitness, etc., or maybe you're just wondering what the heck I've been doing for the past 13 years, since my book, Raw Power!, was originally published.

For those of you who don't know, I was born Stephen Arlin, in Columbus, Ohio in 1969. Shortly after birth, I was taken from my mother and circumcised, vaccinated and given a chemical baby formula to "nourish" me. My first day out of the safety of the womb and, for all intents and purposes, I already had three strikes against me. "Welcome to Planet Earth, little baby boy, this is the way we do things here!"

For the first several years of my life, I ate the Standard American Diet, also known as SAD. My "health food" journey began when I was six. My mother had just finished reading the book "Sugar Blues." In the book, the author argued that refined sugar is an addictive drug and is extremely harmful to the human body. The author concluded that a small dietary change, eliminating refined sugar, makes a huge difference in how good one is able to feel physically and mentally. My mom put this into practice right away in our household. All refined sugar and products which contained this substance were thrown away. Even at the young age of six, I understood what was going on. I would go to the health food store with my mom and watch as she read ingredient labels and researched products. We lived like that for a couple years. Then my parents fell into marital problems and healthy food concerns were abandoned in favor of joint custody and quick trips to fast-food joints.

My next exposure to healthy food wasn't until I was eighteen and a Freshman pitcher for the Arizona State University baseball team. During a game, I looked over at Joe, a fellow pitcher, and he was sitting there in the dugout eating a big bag of raw vegetables. I said to him, "Dude, what the heck are you eating?!" Joe said calmly, "This is what Nolan Ryan eats. He says this is how he gets his heat." "Heat" refers to a pitched ball that's travelling FAST. Nolan Ryan is known as the "Strikeout King" and was entered into the Guinness Book of World Records for the Fastest Pitched Ball. OK, so that was pretty impressive, finding out what Nolan Ryan attributed his unique skill to: the consumption of raw vegetables! I tried it out and I did have a lot more energy and felt stronger, however those were the days of frequent keg parties and a diet of raw vegetables didn't fare well when mixed with gallons and gallons of beer. So, once again, healthy food choices fell by the wayside.

In my early twenties I was into a lot of things one wouldn't consider "mainstream." Whether it was music, politics, philosophy, etc., if something was contrary to what the masses were doing, I'd usually be interested in giving it a look. And that's how I found raw foods. I read my first book about eating a raw-food diet at the end of 1994. I followed that with a book about juicing. From then on, I was hooked. I would never think the same way about food and diet again. I thought to myself, "wow, this is really contrary to society, but also very logical. I'm gonna do it."

I began my raw food journey in January 1995 and, along with two friends, co-founded a hard-hitting "raw foods think-tank" in April of that year. We started out really hard-core and uncompromising, a common trait among twenty-something year-olds. We would set up tables in malls, parks…anywhere, and talk to passers-by about raw foods all day, then go home and have raw food and juicing parties with whoever would show up. Massive Abundance, we called it.

We published our first raw foods book in 1996 and then started a full-time, full-service raw food business…the first of its kind (I later left that company, started Rawpower.com, and the old company was dissolved shortly after).

In 1998, the first edition of Raw Power! was published. I also met my wife, Jolie, that year. As it turns out, it was a mutual interest in raw foods that brought about the good fortune of our paths crossing. Thirteen great years and four awesome kids later, raw foods are still the main focus of our family's diet.

In 2000, shortly after our first child was born, we changed our last name to Bazler (my mother's maiden name). I had always been very close with the Bazler side of the family my whole life, so we decided it was best for our new family to live our lives as Bazlers. Thor was a nickname, so…Thor Bazler. Over the years, some in the raw-food community have been critical of my name change, which I find ridiculous since it was a family decision made for family reasons.

The reason it has taken me so long to update and republish Raw Power! is that over the years, I've gone through a lot of personal growth and attained a lot of new knowledge, and I wasn't sure how I'd be able to weave all this new knowledge into a book that I originally wrote in my twenties, or if I even desired to. I have transformed from that youthful, overzealous, raw-food fanatic into a man/husband/father who doesn't claim to have all the answers anymore. I didn't want to just reprint the old edition and I didn't want to start over with a completely new book either (since there was a lot of good information in the old edition). So, here in your hands is the product of an accumulation of over 15 years of raw food, superfood, and truly natural bodybuilding information.

My favorite books are always the ones from which I learn at least one new, fascinating key principle, idea or "piece of the puzzle" that I can take from that book to add to my life's puzzle, or "spiritual backpack" as my wife calls it. Sometimes, if I'm lucky, I'll find more than one piece. I hope you enjoy this book, and I hope you discover at least one piece for your life's puzzle.

Best wishes!
Thor Bazler

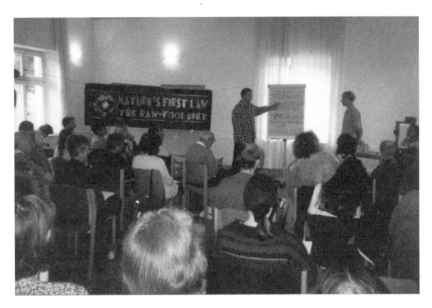

**Thor presents his "Raw Power Seminar"
just outside of Munich, Germany
during a European Tour.**

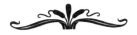

Raw Power

Conversations between healers and patients through the ages.
PATIENT: I have a headache.
HEALER: 2000 B.C. - Here, eat this fruit.
1000 A.D. - That fruit is heathen, say this prayer.
1850 A.D. - That prayer is superstition, drink this potion.
1940 A.D. - That potion is snake oil, swallow this pill.
1985 A.D. - That pill is ineffective, take this antibiotic.
2000 A.D. - That antibiotic is artificial. Here, eat this fruit.

Every living organism on Planet Earth is naturally a raw-food eater. There are trillions of organisms and creatures on this planet that are thriving and living virtually disease-free eating 100% raw foods. There is only one organism that tampers with its food—the human organism. *Trillions to one!* Those are staggering odds. That would make the likelihood that we should be eating our food in a cooked state about 100,000 times more improbable than winning the lottery. You don't want to bet against those kinds of odds, right?

I know raw-food enthusiasts all over the world, in just about every country. I have met raw-foodists that live in inner cities; I have met raw-foodists that live in tropical paradises. The point is, no matter where you live, no matter what condition you live in, you can make the change and eat a lot more raw foods— every living organism on this planet does it, and so can you.

Most health-seekers give up on a raw-food diet (or a high

percentage raw-food diet, 80% plus) when their weight drops and the peer criticism and self-doubt begins. This book is designed to help you reach the next level, to surpass the negativity, and to build a body filled with super-strength and energy!

When you first adopt a raw-food diet, you will lose weight. It is inevitable. After years of eating cooked, processed, dead foods, your body becomes loaded with toxic material. For example, the only way to clean a bathtub filled with dirty water is to pull out the plug and let it completely drain. Once the body has a chance to unload poisons, it will do so. Each organ will cleanse itself, every tissue will purge dead material. The body will detoxify. This is always accompanied by weight loss. "The good will push out the bad."

This detoxification process is the major barrier to achieving a 100% raw-food diet, especially if you are advanced in years. Cooked food clogs up your body and stops detoxification, so to properly detoxify, you must combat cooked-food addiction. Get the cooked food out, bring the raw food in! How do you clean up the river as long as the chemical plant is dumping waste into it upstream?

Do you remember the concept of diffusion from chemistry class? Molecules move from areas of greater concentration to areas of lesser concentration. As the blood thins out on a raw-food diet, toxic, undigested molecules trapped in the lymph will pour into the bloodstream.

As one keeps rinsing, washing, and cleaning the membranous tract, one may experience recurring symptoms of past illnesses. Coughs, colds, headaches, mucus eliminations, diarrhea, sore throats, fevers, rashes, pains that float from one part of the body to another, and the negative mental states of anxiety, depression, and imbalance, may reappear as one persists with a natural lifestyle of raw foods, exercise, and sunshine. Your weight will fall.

To win through, you must endure these discomforts, even if you have to relive (for short periods of time) old sicknesses experienced as far back as your childhood. The toxins and wastes responsible for old sicknesses, which may have lain dormant since infancy, will be released from their hiding places. You may even taste a medicine you ingested years back, or have a craving for a food you have not eaten in decades. I have suddenly tasted breakfast cereals not eaten in twenty-five years!

The cycles of purge and replenishment may last weeks, months, or even a couple of years. It all depends on your lifestyle before. It depends on how toxic your body is. Everybody goes through a different detoxification process. *Embrace the detoxification process, accept it, and get past it.*

During the detoxification period and the initial stages of raw eating, you can and should exercise the muscles and strengthen the body. While exercising, you may experience light-headedness and other detoxification symptoms. You may not feel as strong, because your body is using all of its energy to cleanse and rebuild itself. Always do what you can, where you are, with what you have. Start walking and build up from there if that's what it takes.

You will not put on healthy weight until the body is sufficiently cleansed. Again, this may take a couple of months for some people or a couple of years for others, depending on age and the toxic condition of the body. In my case, I lost 51 pounds (23 kg) initially. I dropped from 238 pounds (107 kg) to 187 pounds (84 kg) and stayed at that weight for 4-5 months when I was transitioning. Then I quickly gained 15 pounds back (6.8 kg) (by exercising and eating the exact same raw-food diet I was eating when I was losing weight), and steadily gained healthy, muscular weight after that.

Anyone can gain all the strength, lean muscle, and healthy weight they want, in any part of the body they choose. If you gain just one wholesome pound per month, in one year, you will gain 12 pounds (5.5 kg)!

Look at your body in the mirror. Look for challenging areas. Exercise where you need development. The areas of your body you consider to be thin or underweight are the areas upon which you should focus your attention and energy.

On a raw-food diet (or high-raw diet), it is easy to gain muscle and unleash a hidden strength and potential if you persist past the negativity and peer pressure. No great success is possible without persistence. Change your peer group if necessary. Get away from toxic, negative people. Water seeks its own level, and you can rest assured that unhappy (or jealous) people will try to bring you down to their level.

It's definitely not an overnight transformation, although you can start to see results immediately. You obviously can't expect to be in perfect physical shape by working out one time. The same is true with anything, for that matter. Fundamentals practiced daily and consistently produce results.

To gain strength and healthy, muscular weight, you must do all you can of the following:

1. think abundantly and powerfully!
2. eliminate artificial substances, drugs and medicines
3. regularly work out with weights
4. get adequate sunshine on the skin
5. maintain your emotional poise

6. be free of toxic environments and mass media
7. get adequate sleep
8. meditate
9. consume enough calories and protein
10. stay hydrated

      Being healthy is our normal and natural state. Being unhealthy is unnatural, and is a direct result of living and eating   . unnaturally.

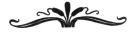

Power of the Mind

If you have the belief that you can do it,
you shall surely acquire the capacity to do it,
even if you do not have it at the beginning.

Human potential is unlimited. There is no point where your memory is too good, your creativity too high, your thought process too clear, your intuition too strong, or your extra sensory too powerful—there is no ceiling! The human mind is amazing.

Health is a composite of a number of factors. The most important factor in attaining the physique that you desire is power of the mind, or attitude. Whoever said that "attitude is everything" was exactly right. Have you heard of the "Self-Fulfilling Prophecy?" If you truly believe something, it is more likely to come true. If you make a concerted effort to gain muscle and healthy weight, you can do it. You must conclusively decide that you *want* to gain strength and weight and make it your number one priority. Write down your goal weight and physique on paper (in your journal, if you have one). To achieve your goal, a vision of the peak is needed, for the first step depends on the last. Imagine or picture your body as it will look when you achieve your goal.

When the going gets tough, it is always the mind that fails first, not the body. What you think about comes about. Closely monitor the conversations and pictures you allow to fill your mind.

Affirm in your own mind, "I am strong; I am powerful; I am unstoppable; I can gain strength and healthy, muscular weight each day." Look at yourself in the mirror and emotionally tell yourself "You cannot be stopped; You are energized; You are unlimited." This is the mindset of a winner. Do you think Olympic athletes beat themselves up daily with their own thoughts? No way! Winners first become winners in their minds. They affirm their own capabilities daily, either in their conscious mind, out loud, on paper, or all three. You must do the same. As long as you are thinking "I am weak," you will be weak. Weak thoughts lead one to progressively identify with weakness. Challenge yourself, use your mind to strengthen your determination, strength, and resolve.

Remember:

- Do it, never doubt it.
- One doubt, and you're out.
- If at first you don't succeed, try again!
- Life is a roller coaster, not a merry-go-round, so hang in there!

The notion that incredible strength and healthy weight cannot be built on a regime of mainly raw foods and superfoods is simply that... a notion. A notion that has absolutely no basis in fact. The 200-pound (91-kg) body of the orangutan, the 500-pound (227-kg) body of the gorilla, and the 3,000-pound (1,364-kg) body of the elephant are all constructed of 100% raw plant food. I am here to settle your mind and show you that great size and strength can be accomplished naturally by humans too.

You have the potential to create the exact body you want. You can restructure and rejuvenate your body by rethinking yourself, by grasping on to a wider vision of yourself. De-program your old thought habits and re-program yourself for mind mastery. Send down a different body plan to your subconscious mind through affirmations and pictures of your ideal self. With consistency, your body and experience will follow suit.

As you engage in vigorous exercise, leverage your mind by focusing or meditating on your strength and physique goals. Do not allow yourself to be distracted. Listen to high-energy music that you like while training.

Anchor and maintain a powerful belief system. The most important pre-requisite for accomplishing any goal and for becoming a vibrant, powerful person is a powerful, undiminished belief that what you are doing is indeed the best way to live. This belief must be the product of your own conclusions. It must be strong enough to carry you through the cyclical lows in the process of attaining your goal. Chance, destiny, and fate cannot circumvent, hinder, or control the firm resolve of the determined. We know nothing until intuition agrees.

Whatever you do, don't do it halfway. Half-measures never have and never will achieve the desired results.

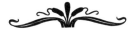

A Raw-Food Diet

*A raw-foodist is not something you become,
it is something that you already are.*

There is a lot of conflicting information in the world today, especially in the field of nutrition. However, there is one thing that is certain: every living organism on Planet Earth is designed to nourish themselves with raw nutrition, and humans are certainly no exception. Every single natural organism on the planet eats exclusively raw foods. No free-living creature ever tampers with its food. Some people consider a raw-food diet the next step past a vegetarian or vegan diet, but it really transcends all diets. It is simply the natural way to nourish your body.

One of the most important elements of health is what we eat. Of course food isn't everything, but it really is the foundation upon which everything else is built. Everything that you physically are right now was once the food that went into your mouth, the air you breathed, the water you drank, etc. Other important factors in health are: positive thoughts and associations, empowering relationships, exercise in nature, sunshine on the skin, interaction with animals, clean air, unpolluted water, and the avoidance of mass media, technology addiction, and social networking addiction. (The Information Age, in many ways, has become overbearing and obsolete. Listening to and acting upon your own body's natural instincts, desires, and needs is the way to health.)

What we eat deeply and radically affects how we think, feel, and behave. In fact, it directly affects how we interact with our planet. Switching to an all raw or high raw-food diet has a profound, positive impact on the environment, as well as ourselves. The principle I am describing here is very simple: life change comes from the inside out; once you change on the inside, everything changes on the outside. To quote my wife: "Begin within."

Cooked Foods

So, what's all the fuss about raw foods versus cooked foods? Eating a diet of mostly cooked carbohydrates, dead proteins, and burned fats, can lead to an internal accumulation of numerous mutagenic (carcinogenic) products caused by the cooking process.

Cooked foods can act malignantly by exhausting your bodily energies, inhibiting your healing process, and decreasing your alertness, efficiency, and productivity. When you treat food with thermal fire, you destroy the life-force in it. The heat of cooking destroys vitamins, enzymes, nucleic acids, chlorophyll, de-animates minerals, and damages fats, turning them into dangerous trans-fatty acids. These changed fats are incorporated into the cell wall and interfere with the respiration of the cell, causing an increase in cancer and heart disease. The heat disorganizes the protein structure, leading to a deficiency of the amino acids. The fibrous or woody element of food (cellulose) is changed completely from its natural condition by cooking. When this fibrous element is cooked, it loses its broom-like quality to sweep the alimentary canal clean.

Fire destroys, it doesn't create anything. When you add flame to something, it becomes less than it was before. If you don't believe me, try adding flame to a piece of paper. Will it become more or less than it was before? Well, the same holds true regarding your food. If you add heat or flame to it, it will become less than it was before. The ramifications of cooking are many.

Eating a diet of mostly (or all!) cooked foods suppresses the immune system. After eating cooked foods, the blood immediately shows an enormous increase of leukocytes, or white blood cells/corpuscles. The white blood cells are supposedly a first line of defense and are, collectively, popularly called "the immune system." This spontaneous multiplication of white corpuscles always takes place in normal blood immediately after the introduction of any virulent infection or poison into the body since the white corpuscles are the fighting organisms of the blood. Conversely, there is no multiplication of white corpuscles when raw plant food is eaten. The constant daily fight (hourly fight for some gluttons!) against the toxic effects of cooked food unnecessarily exhausts the body's strength and vitality, thus causing disease and decreased quality of life.

Ingesting cooked food allows inorganic minerals to enter the blood, circulate through the system, settle in the arteries and veins, and deaden the nerves. After decades of overeating cooked foods, the body loses its flexibility, arteries lose their pliability, nerves lose their power of conveying expressions, the spinal cord becomes hardened, and the tissues throughout the body contract. In many cases, this dead matter is deposited in the various joints of the body, causing enlargement of the joints. In other cases, it accumulates as concretions in one or more of the internal organs, finally accumulating around the heart valves. A lack of flexibility in any area of life, especially in the physical body, causes premature aging and weakness. (The importance of stretching the body and returning the tissues to a natural elasticity cannot be overstated.)

Raw Foods

Raw plant food provides us with more strength, stamina, and energy because it has the best balance of water, nutrients, and fiber, which precisely meet the body's needs.

On a raw-food diet, the mind (memory and the power of concentration) will be clearer. One will be more sharp and alert, and think more logically. Raw foods not only allow us to build a real base of healthy strong muscle tissue, they also allow us to focus more clearly, especially when exercising.

Raw foods will not leave a person with a tired feeling after a meal. There is a tendency toward lethargy after a cooked meal. When eating raw foods, one requires less total sleep and will experience more restful sleep. This allows more time to achieve goals and enjoy exercise activities with family and friends.

Raw foods are easily digested, requiring only 12-24 hours for transit time through the digestive tract, as compared to 36-100 plus hours for some cooked foods. Prolonged digestion creates putrefaction and disease in the colon. It robs the body of energy which could be directed towards gaining strength. Remember, digestion takes by far more energy than any other internal bodily activity.

On a raw-food diet many experience the elimination of body odor and halitosis (bad breath). Eating raw can also alleviate allergies because cooked foods irritate the delicate, thin mucus lining in the body and sinuses. Eating raw can allow space for free-breathing and a better internal environment for vigorous physical training.

Raw foods are delectable, delightful, and delicious and

have more flavor than cooked foods. Cooked food is bland—that is why people need to doctor-up cooked food with loads of sodium and ridiculous additives. These "flavor-enhancing" (excitotoxin) additives irritate your digestive system and overstimulate other organs. Avoid the following harmful additives: refined sugar, table salt, artificial flavors and colors, hydrogenated oil and other suspicious ingredients.

Nature clearly demonstrates, in the eating habits of every form of life, the basic principles of nutrition. Animals, in their feeding, obtain a balanced intake of basic food components so that the ratio of sugars, fats, proteins, carbohydrates, mineral salts, and vitamins to each other remains basically the same.

The plant is the basis of all animal life on Earth; all animals derive their food either directly or indirectly from plants. Eat raw, fresh, organic fruits and vegetables to supply the requisite vitamins and minerals. Eating these will minimize digestive stress and conserve bodily energy. A minimum of digestive power should be expended in order to obtain a maximum of nutritional return. Again, eat only those foods which you can most readily digest and assimilate.

Percentages

If you are interested in trying a 100% raw-food diet (or a high raw diet), you will be eating mostly fruits and smoothies for breakfast, and salads, vegetables, nuts, seeds, avocados, olives, and oils for lunch and dinner. (An extra protein/superfood smoothie at night would be beneficial too to help put on more lean muscle and get more calories in.)

There are different things you can eat in addition to the above fruits, vegetables, salads, smoothies, etc., as most people, for one reason or another, do not stay on a strict 100% raw vegan diet for long (one year or more). Most people are able to stay on an 80% plus raw vegan diet long term, and the other 20% really depends on personal choice.

So, which cooked foods *can* be a healthful addition to a mostly raw diet (especially after all of the above information indicating against cooked food)? For some people, it can mean organic brown rice and steamed veggies. For non-vegans it may mean wild sockeye salmon and organic wild rice. As long as you keep your non-raw choices highly healthy, you'll do great.

There are many different healthy ways to eat and I no longer advocate only a long-term 100% raw vegan diet for everyone. I don't profess to know what every single person on Earth should be eating (though I admit, when I was younger and naive I did!). However, I do know what has worked for me and thousands of others who have ventured down the raw food path.

A good guideline is to try to eat 80-100% fresh, organic, ripe, raw plant foods. I think the best way to think about what foods to eat is this: you want to be eating the most unharmful, most nutrient-rich foods. Period. It's smart to aim high, yes, but don't think that you're failing if you are eating 80% raw and making pretty decent choices with the other 20%. It doesn't have to be all or nothing. You can have times of all raw. I know many people who eat this way and they lead happy, healthy lives.

A 100% raw-food diet is, without a doubt, a life-transforming tool, and I recommend that people at least give it a try for a time. In our present society, not many people could have the discipline to eat an all-raw or high-raw diet if there wasn't something going on biologically (in other words, if there wasn't a "rightness" to it). We are not really human beings, we are human becomings, because we are constantly becoming something more, and the most valuable aspect of 100% raw-foodism is its transformative value. You're not the same person just a little bit healthier. You become a *radically* new person with new interests, goals, and aspirations.

What percentage of raw food should each person eat? Just as the best exercise is the one you will do regularly and joyfully, the same thing goes with a healthy diet. Eat the percentage you will do regularly and joyfully. Think of your raw food journey as "adding in" instead of "taking away." It's human nature that you will revert back to eating unhealthy foods if you see your diet as taking away. Vacillating between a 100% raw vegan diet and binging on cooked food (or junk food!), then fasting, etc. can be very detrimental. (And I've seen this over and over with those who really want to make a 100% raw diet work, but it isn't working, so they binge and then cycle back to raw foods... and all the while they have a lot of guilt and weirdness about their food and themselves.)

Quality of life and health depends on a lot more than just an ideology of health. Enjoying what you eat and feeling satisfied on a daily basis are very important too. There are many really delicious, healthful non-raw foods that, when you add it all up, probably make little or no difference in your overall health.

One key principle of health I've found to be undeniably true over the years is that more important than what you're eating is what you're not eating, especially in today's world of quick and easy convenience foods. In fact, the best thing about eating raw, organic foods is not that they are "magical," but that you are not eating the junk that the majority of people are eating! Raw foods are special, yes, but they are not a cure-all. Eating raw food all by itself won't completely improve your life, but it's a great start. The art of being wise is knowing what to overlook!

Eat the foods you like; eat foods that agree with you.

Since everyone is a bit different, everyone should eat a bit differently, according to their natural instincts, desires, environments, and levels of activity. Eat only foods which you feel satisfy your nutritive needs, digestibility, and assimilation. What is desirable for you may not be desirable for someone else.

Detoxifying

What we must understand and accept is that for every disciplined effort in life, there are multiple rewards. I've seen people go through very mild detoxifications, and I've seen some pretty hard-core detoxifications. It really depends on how you lived your life before. Someone who was a heavy drug user, medicine taker, or smoker is obviously going to have a heavier detoxification than someone who lived their life more in accordance with the laws of nature.

The laws of nature are there for us to use to our benefit. Human progress through knowledge has been solely and exclusively a chiselling away at the distinctions which define the laws of nature. The greatest insights in history have been by those people who revealed a new distinction about nature (which was actually there all along).

When the body gets buried in unprocessed residues of cooked foods and finally has the energy to release them, it will. *There is no magic pill, only a magic process.* As we untangle ourselves out of the cooked-food residues, we release suppressed toxins and emotions. Hang in there, understand what is happening, stay active, get outdoors, and enjoy the abundance life has to offer! Don't worry about detoxification symptoms, they are clear signals that your body is healing.

Remember, you have to detoxify *all* the toxic waste and poisons out of your body, and keep them out, before you can build up on raw foods. You have to be willing to detoxify *all* the way. Again, you can't clean up the river as long as the chemical plant is dumping waste upstream! Our bloodstreams are our most important rivers. It is possible to gain muscle and unleash strength you never knew you had if you simply adhere to the laws of nature.

Be extremely cautious of medications. Medications are poisons and the body must go through a tremendous internal crisis to eliminate and detoxify them. A "poison" is anything ingested that cannot be metabolized and utilized effectively by the body, and that the body must waste resources (greater than any benefit received therefrom) on eliminating and/or detoxifying.

Fasting is the fastest way to heal the body. A good guideline is to fast (drink pure water only) one day a month. Giving your body a rest (from work, workouts and stress) one day a week is also great. Newcomers to the raw-food diet need not worry about fasting until they have been on a high-raw diet for at least six months. It is best to educate yourself first on the subjects of raw-food diet and fasting and take one step at a time, initially just stopping the intake of unhealthy food and progressing from there.

Eating for the Wrong Reasons

A major problem that most people have is eating for emotional reasons. Never eat until you are hungry. Every cell and part of your body must be exercised before you eat so that the food you eat will be properly metabolized. Create a demand for the food every time you eat. <u>Earn your food</u>. Even if you put the best food in your body when you are not hungry, the food will not be assimilated at the most efficient level and it will drain energy unnecessarily.

Here are some good guidelines to keep in mind:

1. Do not eat when fatigued; instead drink only water.
2. Do not eat immediately before beginning exercise.
3. Do not eat when under mental or physical distress.
4. Do not eat when ill.
5. Do not eat junk foods.
6. Do not overeat.
7. Do not eat foods containing pesticides.
8. Do not eat unnatural additives, chemicals and/or other synthetic products.

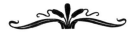

Building Strength and Muscle
with Raw Foods

When I first experimented with eating a 100% raw-food diet, I shed 51 unwanted, unhealthy pounds (238 to 187—I'm 6'2") and then gained back more than 50 pounds of healthy, solid muscle through the unique training workouts and diet ideas outlined in this book.

People may ask, can you gain strength and muscle without eating meat? Just ask vegetarian Bill Pearl, who won four Mr. Universe bodybuilding titles. Arnold Schwarzenegger once said, "Bill Pearl never talked me into becoming a vegetarian, but he did convince me that a vegetarian could become a champion bodybuilder."

You most certainly can build muscle on a plant-based diet, especially if you engage in rigorous anaerobic exercise. This is how to build muscle mass. It is funny that people believe you can build muscle out of cooked, processed animal muscle, but not on fruits and green-leafed vegetables. Cooked-eating, meat-worshipping, pill-popping, steroid-injecting bodybuilders have artificial strength. They have truly accepted a Faustian bargain (a short-term gain at the expense of a long-term tragedy). Sooner or later, they will have to pay the price. And they do, as we see with most of the retired bodybuilders and athletes whose bodies have fallen apart by the time they reach the age of fifty.

Also, what is known to the world as "Natural Bodybuilding" is hardly natural at all. Just because someone

trains steroid-free, it doesn't mean they are building a natural
body. Food is the foundation of everything we are physically. If
you are eating unnatural and harmful food, you are engaged in
"Unnatural Bodybuilding."

The only way to truly build your body is through eating
naturally, and in a balanced way. It has been noted that all long-
term raw-foodists eat out of the following classes of foods:

1. Green-Leafy Vegetables and Algaes (such as
   chlorella and spirulina, Thor's Hammer)
2. High-Water-Content Sugar Fruits (melons,
   tropical/subtropical fruits, etc.)
3. Fats (avocados, coconuts, nuts, seeds,
   olives, durians, etc.)

These three food classes form the essentials of a raw-food
diet. These foods balance against each other and keep you centered. Think of the three food classes as corners of a triangle, the
center being the balance point. For example, when one eats too
many fatty foods, the internal propensity (or instinct) is to eat
more greens and juicy sugar fruits to balance. If one eats too
many juicy sugar fruits, the internal propensity (or instinct) is to
eat more greens and fats to balance. If one eats too many greens,
the internal propensity (or instinct) is to eat more fats and juicy
sugar fruits to balance. Keep this in mind as you develop a consistent raw-diet which can catapult you to your maximum potential.

Chlorophyll-rich foods are the blood of life. The chloro-
phyllous green, leafy vegetables and algaes are the richest
sources of alkaline mineral salts, living carbohydrates, and top-
quality proteins. The most complex laboratory in the world
resides in the photosynthetic green-leaf organs of plants. The

leaves contain an excess of organic base compounds in a colloidal form.

For maximum strength and bodybuilding, include a large green-leafy salad in your diet each day. Organic or home-grown romaine lettuce or dinosaur kale are two of the most superior leafy-vegetables nutritionally and they are the most palatable when eaten alone. Also use the chlorophyll-rich and mineral-saturated wild greens such as dandelion, malva (mallow), lamb's quarters, thistle, etc. The more natural your food, the better. Also, celery (the favorite food of the gorilla) is a fine addition to the bodybuilder's diet. Celery provides organic sodium which balances out the potassium of fruits, providing a balanced internal chemistry. Cut up an apple or an avocado and mix it with your salad if you find it dry.

Chlorella and spirulina are superfood algaes that play an enormous role in my daily diet. These highly-beneficial superfoods are two of the purest natural green foods known to humankind. I designed a product that I call "Thor's Hammer," which consists of a special blend of pure chlorella and pure spirulina and I discuss this product in more detail later on in this book.

Fruits are in many ways our most natural food. Try to eat mostly non-hybridized fruit (fruit with viable seeds) and wild fruit. I do not buy into the "hypoglycemia is caused by fruit" idea, even if it is hybridized commercial fruit. I do believe, from experience, that a good percentage of the fruits you eat should be non-sweet fruits such as cucumber, red bell pepper, tomato, corn, and zucchini. I also believe that fruit causes a cleansing of refined sugars out of the body which may have been stored there for years, even decades. Never eat refined sugar of any kind (that includes the sugar found in bread and other cooked starches). Find one or more staple fruits which you like so much, they make you feel as if you can live off of them alone. I personally prefer berries, melons and citrus fruits.

Though it is not totally necessary, for ideal digestion, eat one type of fruit at a time. Try not to mix different types of fruits together. Many people I know follow a "mono-diet" when eating fruit. Eat fruits that are in season (see the Seasonal Produce Availability section later in this book), and regularly eat heavy fuel or "high-calorie" fruits such as apples, avocados, bananas, cherimoyas, dates, durians, grapefruits, lemons, mangos, etc.

Nuts are also a potent food, especially in the winter season. I do not like to use the word "moderation," but remember to moderate with nuts. You can get "nutted out." Eat nuts with naturally-dried fruits for superior digestion. My experience has shown that eating dried fruits and nuts in the winter increases one's resistance to cold weather. Nuts are a heavy food which can provide you with the fuel or calories for long, intense workouts.

To gain strength and healthy weight, I also recommend sending "hot" food through the intestinal tract on a regular basis. Pick your favorite hot raw foods, whether they be: garlic, onions, ripe hot peppers, ginger, radishes, etc. You can juice these foods with vegetables or mix them with salads. Hot foods burn out parasites and stimulate the intestines. (I have noted that with some people turning on to raw foods, excessive thinness is often associated with parasite infestations.)

Protein is a heavy building material which appears in nuts, seeds and algaes, but is also available in vegetables and even fruits. Cooked proteins can clog the tissue system causing the muscle tissue to puff up. Strength is gained at the expense of vitality and the body is put under a tremendous strain to prevent damage to the ligaments and joints. Adequate, raw proteins help you to gain desirable muscular weight, there's no doubt about it, but are not necessary in the ridiculously large amounts recommended by commercial bodybuilding "experts."   .

The gorilla is the strongest land mammal pound-for-pound. A gorilla has the strength equivalent to bench pressing 4,000 pounds (1800 kg)! Gorillas eat primarily green-leafy materials, which are the real body builders. Of course, the gorilla is a 100% raw plant eater! Do you think if a gorilla ate fast food, candy, donuts, sodapop, etc. every day it would be able to perform feats of strength like this? I think not.

Raw proteins are built from substances called amino acids. Of the 22 necessary amino acids, there are eight which our bodies must get from outside sources. All of these eight are present in raw plant foods (especially in green foods) in their correct proportions. Think of a cow which is 1,000 plus pounds (450 kg) of protein flesh. What does a cow eat? Grass. All the amino acids necessary for the cow to build an enormous body are present in grass, and any green plant for that matter.

Remember, a cooked food diet drains and dehydrates your body of precious, heavy, living water. Living water is derived most abundantly from living plants, especially fruit. Living water is not just filtered water which comes through the roots and into the plant; living water is actually created during photosynthesis. Living water is heavier, more electrified, and has greater solubility properties than ordinary water (the hydrogen atoms are pulled together more tightly in each molecule of living water, thus giving the molecule greater polarity).

Living water weighs more on a molecular level than dead tap or spring water (the 60 trillion cells multiplied by the slightly heavier water-weight of every molecule produces a big difference in overall body weight). When a diet consists of a high percentage of cooked foods, the water stored in one's body goes towards diluting and digesting the dry, enzyme-less foods and a person feels drained.

Also, as a general rule, the higher the water-content of the food, the higher its energy and vibration. The lighter your diet, the more energy you will have. To achieve your desired weight, stabilize the living-water weight level in your body. One's living-water weight will more stabilize the closer one's diet is to 100% raw.

Dead food, negative emotions, and inactivity drain your energy and cause weight loss. This becomes definitely more true the closer you get to a 100% raw diet. My experience has indicated that one cannot reach her/his ideal body weight unless the body is significantly purified by a high raw-diet.

Listed below are three special strategies I have successfully employed to gain healthy, muscular weight over the years. Employ them as part of your daily dietary regime and you will see results.

Strategy 1: Raw Power! Smoothies and Thor's Hammer

A while back, I developed a line of all-raw, vegan, certified organic, 100% pure smoothie blends called Raw Power! Protein Superfood Blends. These Protein Superfood blends are designed to be blended into smoothies with raw, fresh or frozen fruits, superfood powders and juice. Always strive to use fresh, raw, organic ingredients.

In a base of fresh orange juice, coconut water, or nut milk, I blend two or three organic bananas, 2-3 scoops of Raw Power! Protein Superfood powder, one cup frozen, organic berries (blueberries or raspberries are my favorites), a handful of organic goji berries, and a tablespoon of a dark green superfood powder (such as Vitamineral Green). Try these smoothies yourself.

Then, depending on your tablet-swallowing capabilities, with each swig of your smoothie, take 3-15 Thor's Hammer tablets. Thor's Hammer consists of pressed tablets of pure broken-cell-wall chlorella and pure spirulina. No fillers or binders are used, so the tablets disintegrate rather quickly when consumed. The tablets work great because you can enjoy the wonderful taste of your smoothie without every swig tasting like chlorella and spirulina. Remember to start with a small amount of the Thor's Hammer tablets at first and build up slowly over time. This smoothie contains approximately 25-40 grams of protein (depending on amount of Thor's Hammer tablets taken) and little to no fat, and is bristling with health benefits.

Strategy 2: Coconuts and green juice

I have also used the following formula to help energize my blood, build my body, and gain several pounds of healthy muscular weight:

I buy young coconuts which are commonly found in Asian-food markets. (Young coconuts are now also becoming easier to find in the produce section of many health food stores — if your health food store doesn't carry them yet, just ask!) I open the coconut and pour the water into a pitcher. I then scoop out the soft, jelly-like pulp for myself or my family, or save it for smoothies or my wife's coconut custard. I add freshly-made green juice to the coconut water, which saturates my body with usable muscle-building minerals.

This program targets the blood specifically. When you rebuild your blood, you rebuild your body. Coconut water is the closest substance to human blood plasma found in the plant

world. Fifty-five percent of the blood is plasma. Green chlorophyll is the closest substance to human hemoglobin in the plant
world. Coconut water combined with green juice is a powerhouse way to revitalize the blood and build the body. Ann
Wigmore often recommended coconut water mixed with wheatgrass juice, a combination I enjoy as well.

I eat the pulp inside the coconut for its incredible raw
plant fat content. Raw plant fats, as I mentioned before, are
essential to a powerfully vibrant raw diet. Healthy fats are as
important in the human diet as protein is. Raw plant fats lubri-
cate the digestive tract, they are "soft" on the body (easy to
assimilate), and they deliver specific protection to the wall of
each cell. Fats also provide extra electrons to the cells and thus
they are an anti-oxidant.

Here is one of my secret raw bodybuilding formulas:

Captain's Powerhouse

In a blender:
1 young coconut (juice and pulp)
1 large avocado
2 handfuls of wild or organic greens

Strategy 3: Eat only once or twice a day.

Eating only once or twice a day is another strategy you
can employ to gain strength and muscular weight. Eat large
meals when you eat. Note: This is not necessarily the optimal
way for everyone to eat, but keep in mind what your goal is
here—to gain strength and healthy, muscular weight. After you
achieve your desired strength and weight, you can return to a
more sustainable eating schedule.

An example of this principle can be seen in Sumo Wrestlers. While they are obese and unhealthy, the way they eat to gain weight is interesting and instructive. Many Sumo Wrestlers fast all day and then, right before they go to bed, they eat a massive meal, consisting largely of dense, rich cooked foods. What happens is the body "thinks" there is a shortage of food all day so it conserves energy and the metabolism slows way down. Then, they eat a massive meal right before they go to sleep and the body is not able to process and assimilate most of the food—so they inevitably gain weight (of course not healthy weight!). It has been my experience that raw-foodists who eat all day are thinner than those who eat once or twice a day. For raw-eaters who eat all day, their bodies sense that there is an abundance of food so their metabolism speeds up in order to process all the food coming in.

To further illustrate this concept, I will use the following analogy: Anyone familiar with standard weight-training principles knows that to build mass you need to do low-repetition exercises with a heavy weight (1-30 reps). And to tone-up, you need to do high-repetition exercises with a light weight (30-100 reps). The same principles can be applied to eating for mass or eating to tone-up. High-repetition exercises with a low weight equates to eating a high frequency of small meals throughout the day. You are not able to gain much mass by eating this way. Low-repetition exercises with a high weight equates to eating a low frequency of large meals during the day (only one or two meals a day). This is a key aspect of gaining weight and strength on a raw-food diet.

Many years ago, I took a 12-day trip to Hawaii. There were so many exotic fruits there, I found myself eating pretty much all day (high frequency of small meals). Guess what? I lost 13 pounds in those 12 days. When I returned home, I ate only at night, stayed hydrated with pure water, lifted weights and took in sunlight during the day and the weight returned quickly.

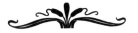

Protein:

How Much is Enough?

Several years ago, I bought into the "protein isn't that important, you can get enough from raw fruits and vegetables" dogma in the raw-food community. I even wrote about it in articles and in the past editions of Raw Power! That was until I witnessed an incredible feat of strength and endurance in front of Whole Foods Market in San Diego. A friend I worked with told me about the guy in the story below, and then I happened to see him for myself. At the time, it seemed like I was just in the right place at the right time, but now I know it was meant to be.

Near the dining patio in front of the store, there was a crowd gathering around a well-built man in his 40s. He was challenging people to a strength contest. In fact, not only was he challenging a person at a time, he was challenging "any ten of you against me." Meaning, he was saying that he could outlift the COMBINED efforts of any ten people in the audience. I thought to myself, "Ok, this will be worth watching. In fact, I'll participate. Hey, I'm the Raw Power guy, I have to participate!" So a few of us men stepped forward, and then a couple more—only five guys total, but all of us were young, in good shape and worked out regularly with weights. The man said, "ok, you five do your lifts, add them all up, then double that number. I'll beat it." The man simply had two 35-pound dumbbells and his guidelines were: "Stand up straight and hold a dumbbell in each hand.

Next, curl both dumbbells up to your shoulders, twist them, then press them up over your head to full extension. Bring them down to your sides again. That is one rep. Keep doing reps until you can't do any more." I knew I could do a bunch of these so I thought, "This will be fun! No way this guy's gonna win this challenge..."

The first of us five challengers went and he only did six reps. The second guy went and he did ten. I went next and I did thirty-nine, which won me a nice round of applause, even from the man challenging us! The last two guys went and they did twelve and fifteen, respectively. We added them up—82. Doubling made the number to beat 164. I thought, "There's no way this guy can do 164 reps, that's ridiculous!"

Well, you know what happened next, right? It was stunning to watch this guy do 165 reps and then stop. He could have kept on going. I could tell he was getting a little tired, but something allowed him to go and go, far past the point of fatigue that the normal bodybuilder could withstand. I just had to ask him what his diet was like. I thought he would start rattling off a bunch of long latin words or something, but he said simply, "Mostly raw-food protein shakes and green vegetable juices." I thought, "Wow, this guy is into raw foods?! And he's actually into protein?!" It was at that moment when I started to re-think how much protein is necessary to build super strength. I also implemented the high-rep "challenge exercise" I had learned that day into my weekly weight training routine, and I still do it two times a week (see Workouts chapter for my detailed routine).

After I witnessed this impressive feat of strength and endurance first hand, I began looking for high-protein sources of raw vegan foods. During my search, I happened across a hemp seed company who was making hemp seed oil from hemp seeds. When hemp seeds are pressed to produce hemp oil, what's left over is the fiber, or "hemp meal," which is very high in protein and very low in fat. The owner of that company asked me if I wanted to test it out. He sent me a few bags to try out. It was amazing stuff. I was making raw food smoothies with it and working out with weights and I was achieving great results. I started sharing it with my friends and customers and they loved it too. This product later became known as "Hemp Protein" and to this day is still a major part of my diet. (And, NO, you will not fail a drug test by eating hemp protein! Hemp and Marijuana are entirely different. There is no THC (the mind-altering substance found in marijuana) in hemp seeds or hemp protein.)

I also started researching the diets of elite athletes, body-builders and trainers. I experimented by emulating the tidbits of dietary knowledge I learned, but I tweaked their ideas around to make even better, healthier choices. (Substituting egg whites in their diets to hemp protein in mine—things like that.)

Three such examples I found of extremely successful and physically fit people were Bruce Lee, Sylvester Stallone and Jack LaLanne. None of these men are (or were) raw-foodists or super-foodists, but we can learn an important lesson by taking a look at one thing they all had in common with the Challenger at Whole Foods: the importance of healthy high-protein drinks in the diet.

Bruce Lee

Joe Weider, the founder of the Mr. Olympia bodybuilding contest, once described Bruce Lee's physique as "the most defined body I've ever seen." Coming from the founder of the Mr. Olympia bodybuilding contest, that's about as good a compliment as one can receive.

Although Lee never developed a diet of his own, we can learn from his books and what his friends and associates have said about the way he ate. Lee avoided empty, refined calories and his diet included protein shakes; he always tried to consume one or two every day. Hmm...if success leaves clues, then there's a big clue right there. The "most defined body" Joe Weider has ever seen was nourished by one or two protein shakes a day. High quality, bio-available protein helps refuel your body and helps to build lean muscle.

Lee also believed in taking the highest-quality supplements he could find (not as easy in the 1960s and 1970s as it is today!) and once said, "Use only that which works, and take it from any place you can find it." Nowadays we have daily access to very high-quality, clean and pure, super healthy protein-rich foods and supplements.

Sylvester Stallone

Hollywood legend Sylvester Stallone is also a big fan of daily morning protein smoothies mixed with fresh fruit. The International Federation of Bodybuilders named him the "Body of the 80s," an amazing honor for a movie star! Usually one would think this title would be given to a professional champion bodybuilder.

Several years ago, I read an article about Stallone's diet and exercise routine. In that article, he said he basically eats the same thing every morning: a protein smoothie and a half cup of oatmeal. He said he is "like a race horse. You eat the same thing, you get a similar kind of performance." Another important clue: doing the same thing on a consistent basis produces great results.

Jack LaLanne

Jack is one of America's original exercise and nutrition gurus. Jack's life was transformed at the age of 15, when he attended a lecture by a nutritionist, who promised Jack that if he gave up junk food and exercised regularly, he could attain great health. Jack took on the challenge with the zeal and tenacity that would become his personal trademarks. He began lifting weights and sought out all the information he could find on human anatomy, bodybuilding, diet, and fitness.

He continued to follow a strict regimen of diet, exercise, and supplementation that helped to keep him youthful into his nineties. Jack once said, "Exercise is king and nutrition is queen: together, you have a kingdom." And, you guessed it, every morning his meal consisted of a protein and fruit smoothie.

*   *   *   *   *

Countless others are also now recommending protein shakes, such as Mixed Martial Arts Ultimate Fighter Champion Ken Shamrock and his Lion's Den of fighters. Ken says, "All of us drink one or two protein shakes a day. They help us build muscle and keep our weight up."

Needless to say, I am now also a big proponent of daily high-protein smoothies, although I take it a few steps further and consume them all raw, organic and vegan. A raw-food, vegan diet is fantastic for slimming and overall health but, to build super strength and muscle mass, extra protein is required. There will undoubtedly be people in the raw-food community who will tell you differently, but it's usually a guy who weighs a-buck-thirty, or a guy who can run a marathon, but has the physique of a thirteen year-old boy. If impersonating a beanpole interests you, then you probably wouldn't be reading this book right now. If super strength and muscle mass interest you like they do me, then please read on.

Over the years, I have found that a person eating a high-raw diet and working out regularly with weights needs about a half a gram of protein per desired pound of bodyweight per day to achieve his or her goal physique. Example: If your goal physique is 200 pounds and ripped, low bodyfat, super strong, etc., then a minimum of 100 grams of usable, absorbable protein per day will be required. Not all protein is created equal—in fact, quality and absorbability can differ greatly amongst protein sources.

A good daily guideline is this: try to consume the highest amount of protein you can with the highest percentage of that protein being raw, organic and vegan. This way, you have a good daily goal and it will be very difficult to overdo protein intake.

The key here is to get plenty of rest and consume the necessary amount of protein so that your muscles repair and grow quickly. As you continue to work out, your metabolism will improve and you'll find that you don't take as long to recover.

After a workout, how much protein is optimal? In a study conducted by Dr. Stuart Phillips and associates, his research found that 20 grams of protein maximally stimulates protein synthesis rates. After 20 grams, there was no further increase in protein synthesis. For example, 40 grams did not stimulate protein synthesis greater than 20 grams.

Here's more on the study... To examine the effect of how different dosages of protein powder affected protein synthesis rates, researchers had young healthy men who had previous resistance training experience perform daily intense resistance exercise and consume a protein drink that contained either 5, 10, 20, or 40 grams of protein. Interestingly, they found that increasing protein intake stimulated protein synthesis in a dose up to 20 grams of dietary protein.

This data suggests that there is a maximal rate at which dietary amino acids can be incorporated into muscle tissue at one time and that with increasingly higher concentrations of amino acids, there is no further stimulation of muscle protein synthesis. So how many times in a day could someone consume such a dose (20 grams) to stimulate muscle anabolism that would ultimately translate into muscle growth? The researchers speculated that 4-6 times daily of 20 grams of protein would be the optimal measure to increase anabolism and increase muscle mass.

The protein content of most protein powders on the market is derived from animal sources like whey (which causes bloating and is really just a waste product of the dairy industry—until someone thought to package and sell it), chemical sources, or highly heated (cooked) sources, and are not highly absorbable or assimilable, as protein powders should be. The protein content of these denatured powders is misleading. A cheap or junky commercial product which boasts of 30 grams of protein per serving is not actually supplying that amount to the body, and even if it were, the body would not reap much benefit, if any, over 20 grams anyway.

Raw, Organic, Vegan Protein Sources and Raw Bodybuilding Supplements

I used to be opposed to taking supplements because of the synthetic nature of them and the fact that the vast majority of them are poor-quality, toxic abominations. Things have since changed and there are now some really good raw, organic bodybuilding supplements on the market today. I have found some of them to be of high-quality, high integrity, and very helpful to the health and strength seeker. What to look for in a healthy protein powder, for instance, is 100% food-based and derived from certified organic raw plant sources and one that is fully absorbable and assimilable.

Raw Power! Protein Superfood Blend was born out of my wife and I wishing such a product existed for our own use. We would talk about how it would be great if there were a 100% organic, 100% raw, 100% vegan, 100% clean, 100% HEALTHY protein powder out there—with no fillers and no average ingredients—strictly the best ingredients planet Earth has to offer.

After a few years of trying dozens of different ingredient blends, I finally got it just perfect—perfect for everyone: men, women, children, young, old, active, less-active, athlete, vegan, vegetarian, whole-food-eater, etc. It is clean, usable nutrition for every body, for everyone who wants to add premium-quality, vegetarian protein and/or super nutrition to their diet. My wife, kids and I make it a part of our mornings. What better way to start our day together than with a healthy, delicious super smoothie full of protein and clean, organic nutrition!

Raw Power! is not just a protein powder, it's a Superfood Blend. In fact, we weren't sure if we should market it as a Protein Powder or Superfood Blend since it's really both. But we realize that a lot of people out there need and want more clean, high-quality protein in their diets, and that's what they look for.

We're proud of this product—it's what we were wishing for and waiting for, and we bet what a lot of people have been waiting for, too!

The all-raw, organic, vegan ingredients are: Hemp Protein Powder, Brazil Nut Protein Powder, Maca, Goji Berry Powder, Mesquite Powder and Maca Extreme (a more potent version of maca). These ingredients have been carefully selected and formulated to produce a natural, balanced, nutrient-rich protein product.

Hemp Protein Powder is a natural protein powder, containing over 50% protein. Hemp Protein Powder is made from hemp seeds, which have the most complete edible and usable protein in the vegetable kingdom. This high-performance protein powder is easily digestible with 65% globulin edestin and 35% albumin protein—more than any other plant!

Brazil Nut Protein Powder contains nearly 50% protein and provides antioxidant benefits with its high selenium content. Traditionally, brazil nuts have been regarded as the most calorie-dense of all vegetarian foods.

Maca Powder is an ancient superfood that was consumed by Incan Warriors to increase strength and endurance. Native Peruvians have traditionally utilized this South American root since pre-Incan times for both nutritional and medicinal purposes. Maca is a wonderful source of natural vital nutrients.

Goji Berry Powder is a naturally-concentrated extract of what is considered by many to be the world's most nutrient-rich fruit—the goji berry (Lycium). Goji berries have been used in traditional Asian medicine for over 5,000 years. Much has been written about the health-promoting properties of this amazing fruit.

Mesquite Powder is a traditional Native American food produced by gathering ripened seed-pods from the mesquite tree and grinding them into a fine high-protein powder (approximately 20% protein). For centuries mesquite has been a source of nutrition for Native Americans and indigenous peoples in the arid regions of the earth.

Maca Extreme is the most potent form of maca in the world. It is produced by juicing freshly-harvested maca roots and then drying the juice at a low temperature into a fine powder. Once it is dried, the powder is sifted so only the finest particles make it through into the final product, which produces a high-nutrient powder.

Other important attributes of Raw Power! Protein Superfood Blend:

NO pesticides
NO cholesterol
NO GMOs
NO added sugar
NO trans fats
NO hydrogenated oil
NO dairy
NO wheat or gluten
NO soy
NO preservatives
NO artificial colors, flavors or ingredients
NO animal residues
NO dyes
NO hormones
NO irradiation

<u>To maximize the benefits from your workout, Raw Power Protein smoothies are best consumed within 30 minutes after your workout</u>.

In the case of sensitivities and/or allergies, some of our customers order the individual ingredients that best fit their needs to make their own protein superfood blends. (Hemp Protein Powder, Maca Powder, Acai Powder, Mesquite Powder, Goji Berry Powder, Brazil Nut Protein Powder, Mangosteen Powder, Camu Camu Powder, etc.) All these ingredients are under the Raw Power brand label, and we only brand the highest-quality products available.

Another fantastic raw, organic bodybuilding product I take every day is such an important part of my diet, I named it <u>Thor's Hammer</u>, after the Norse god Thor's powerful weapon of choice. At a whopping 70% protein content, Thor's Hammer is the perfect combination of two of the world's most powerful foods: pure chlorella and pure spirulina.

Chlorella gets its name from its chlorophyll content (highest of all known plants). It is prized for its high-protein content, many health benefits, and nutrient offerings.

Spirulina is a high-energy, high-protein food, valued for its detoxifying and alkalizing benefits.

Chlorella and Spirulina are each considered by many in the health field as "perfect foods" — so it makes perfect sense to offer them together, in their purest form, in Thor's Hammer!

This is a low-temperature, 100% raw product and consists of pressed tablets of pure broken-cell-wall chlorella and pure spirulina. No fillers or binders are used, so the tablets disintegrate rather quickly when consumed.

I've been taking this product every single day for the last couple years, and what I've found is that I can't believe in all my years of eating raw foods, I didn't give much attention to these amazing foods. I started out with 10-20 tablets per day, and slowly increased the amount every few days; now I'm up to almost 300 per day (which is over 50 grams of protein by itself!). Three-hundred tablets sounds like a high amount, but it's only about 75 grams in terms of weight and actually quite easy to do once your body acclimates to it. I've heard stories of olympic athletes taking 60 grams of chlorella or spirulina a day, and I thought, "WOW, that would be great to be able to build up to that amount." Well, I've done it, and surpassed it.

This new product has had a huge impact on my recent muscle- and strength-building, and overall health—I feel great. What I do is drink a Raw Power Smoothie or glass of organic orange juice in the morning and, with every sip, I'll take around 12-15 tablets. At the end of the smoothie or juice, I've taken well over 100 tablets. That's how I start my day each morning, which I feel, for me, is the most nutritionally superior way possible. Then, throughout the day, whenever I eat anything at all, I'll take a few more small handfuls of tablets, tapering off as it gets later in the day. Then, since they are high-energy foods, I won't take any within a few hours of bedtime. I prefer tablets over powder because if I was taking powder all day, all my food would taste like chlorella/spirulina, and I enjoy a myriad of tastes, so the tablets work perfectly. If you're like me, and love to experiment and find new foods to assist with overall health and strength-building, you're going to love this stuff. Remember to start out small, your body will need time to adjust...believe me!

Protein content of Thor's Hammer:
every 20 tablets = 3.5 grams of protein

Vitamineral Green is one the most nutrient-dense, mineral-rich superfood products ever created. Designed to be taken on a daily basis as part of one's bodybuilding or cleansing program, it contains 100% raw, organic or wildcrafted superfoods, with no fillers, the best probiotic formulation ever put together (designed to implant good bacteria in the intestines), soil organisms, and a full digestive enzyme complex. It is neutral tasting, easily dissolvable and can be added to smoothies and juices.

Vitamineral Green is more like a meal than a supplement, as far as content goes. The mineral density of the foods used in this product is around 24%. A "very high" rating is 17% and average is 8-12%! The dominant mineral in this mix is silica. This was done on purpose because research has shown that silica is actually the most important alkaline mineral and the mineral that seems to be most deficient in the general population and even among raw-foodists. Silica is found predominately in horse-tail, nettles, nopal cactus, dandelions, etc. Silica is very important. It is necessary for building all connective tissue cells, as well as those of the hair, nails and skin.

Spirulina Manna is 65% protein and contains all 8 essential amino acids. Spirulina is the world's highest known plant-source of vitamin B-12 and also includes vitamins A, B-1, B-2, B-6, E, K, chlorophyll, cell salts, phytonutrients, and enzymes. The ancient Aztecs thrived on spirulina from Lake Texcoco in Mexico. Goes great with young coconut juice!

Tocotrienols (Super Vitamin E) — This balanced whole food provides a stable variety of essential nutrients necessary to properly fuel a healthy body. Providing a full protein complement, this raw rice bran whole-food complex is highly beneficial for those who require a boost to their nutritional protocol. Tocotrienols contain vitamins, minerals, and essential fatty acids necessary to enhance health. They are the most potent form of antioxidant vitamin E available and a rich source of B vitamins. Tocotrienols were at one time more than $4,000 a bottle in alternative cancer clinics! (Good for us that they're now very affordable at under $30 per pound.) Great to include in smoothies.

*   *   *   *   *

I always buy and consume the highest quality foods possible. Just as with car shopping, or any kind of shopping for that matter, there is always a quality difference. Rolls Royce vs. Hyundai—yep, there's a difference—a big difference! Beware of cheap, commercial brands and products with ingredient lists that read like a science fiction story. Most products out there are riddled with chemicals, pesticides, and artificial ingredients from mysterious sources. They are made commercially, for mass consumption, and made as cheaply as possible.

Always keep in mind you can eat great protein-rich foods all day, but if you don't work out with weight-bearing or resistance exercises, you will not gain muscle.

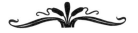

Minerals

*You can trace every sickness, every disease and
every ailment to a mineral deficiency.*
— Linus Pauling

Minerals are essential for all living organisms. Whereas vitamins are organic substances (made by plants, humans or animals), minerals are inorganic elements that come from the soil and water. Animals and humans absorb minerals from the foods they eat and drink. Minerals are nutrients that your body needs to grow and develop normally and have a unique role to play in maintaining our health. They boost the immune system, support growth and development, and help cells and organs do their jobs. Your body needs larger amounts of some minerals, such as calcium, to grow and stay healthy. Other minerals like chromium, copper, iodine, iron, selenium, and zinc are called trace minerals because you only need very small amounts of them each day.

We are made up of minerals. It's really as simple as that. "You are what you eat" is true! A diet high in raw, organic, alkaline minerals is absolutely essential for superior health. A diet lacking in these minerals is disastrous, especially for a bodybuilder.

Often referred to as the "Godfather of Fitness," health, diet and fitness guru Jack LaLanne once said, "I am a huge believer in vitamins and minerals, and even though I eat right, I take supplements as an insurance policy. I take everything, from

A to Z, and it's all from natural sources." Jack lived to the age of 96 and was often seen doing push ups and jumping jacks on the beach well into his 90s. I don't know about you, but I tend to listen to people who have achieved such amazing results in their lifetimes.

Mineral Supplements

There are some who will tell you that you can get all the minerals you need from food. That may be true if one is eating all highly-mineralized wild and organic food grown in highly-mineralized soil away from civilization, pollution and chemicals. But, really, what percentage of people on Earth are doing that? I don't know the exact percentage but I can guess that it's somewhere close to 0%. I used to be one of those "all supplements are unnatural, just eat all raw foods and you'll be fine" people, but that was before I ran into problems myself and started to look into supplementing my diet with some really good high-mineral products. One such product for me has been <u>Vitamineral Green</u> (mentioned in the last chapter). Adding a heaping tablespoon of Vitamineral Green raw superfood to your daily shake or smoothie works wonders! It is raw, organic, and vegan too. The high silicon content, the probiotics, enzymes, and trace minerals of this superfood make it a great muscle and bone builder. A companion product, Vitamineral Earth, is also a fantastic source of concentrated raw, organic bodybuilding minerals. Many people enjoy taking them together to get the whole spectrum of available minerals.

Another great mineral product is <u>Blue Ocean Minerals</u>. It is well known that pure ocean water contains all the known minerals. Using a natural solar process, the maker of Blue Ocean Minerals came up with a way to concentrate all the minerals from pure ocean water from a pristine region of Australia's Great Barrier Reef into a powerful mineral solution, and then reduce the sodium content 98%. One of the things I really like about this product is that the full spectrum of minerals (90 plus minerals and trace elements) is present in its precise natural proportion and balance, compared to other mineral products on the market which contain random quantities and proportions. The minerals which naturally compose our blood mimic the same minerals found in ocean water, which makes ocean-derived minerals perfectly suited for, and most easily absorbed by, the human system. I just add a couple teaspoons of Blue Ocean Minerals to all the ingredients I blend in my morning smoothie, and then I know I'm getting a full spectrum of high-quality minerals, equivalent to four cups of pure ocean water, but without all the sodium!

Methylsulfonylmethane (<u>MSM Powder</u>) is a naturally occurring sulfur compound and nutritional component of many foods. It is found in the normal diets of humans and almost all other animals. MSM is made up of 34% sulfur, the fourth most abundant mineral in the human body. MSM supports healthy, active lifestyles and benefits multiple structures and functions within the body, including connective tissues and the respiratory system. Sulfur is necessary for the structure of every cell in the body. And because the body utilizes and expends it on a daily basis, sulfur must be continually replenished for optimal nutrition and health.

MSM originates in the oceans where microscopic plankton release sulfur compounds into seawater, which is quickly converted to DMS, a volatile sulfur compound that escapes into the atmosphere. In this suspended, gaseous state, the DMS reacts with ozone and ultraviolet sunlight to create DMSO and DMSO2, known as MSM. MSM then falls to the earth with the rain, where it is collected and concentrated in plants and trees. Although MSM is abundant in nature, even the richest natural sources only provide MSM in the level of several parts per million.

Made from the pulp of pine tree and needles, Raw Power MSM is made in the USA and held to strict product specifications, making it the highest quality and most consistent MSM available on the market.

People frequently ask me if I take a daily multivitamin. Well, I take Thor's Hammer tablets every day, which have so much nutrition, and so many benefits, that I consider them my "daily multi" of sorts, but I also sometimes take a multivitamin called <u>Vita Synergy</u>. It's the highest-quality multi I've found and Vita Synergy has separate formulas for men and women, which I think is very important. Another good choice is a multivitamin called <u>Raw One</u>, which also has separate formulas for men and women.

Sodium

The importance of natural sodium for health seekers and bodybuilders cannot be overstated. I recently watched a program in which they did a profile on a popular bodybuilder who said he eats pickles for sodium. Raw olives contain a good natural sodium content, are the fruit highest in minerals, and are a much better choice than pickles (specifically <u>Raw Power Kalamata Olives</u>—they contain celtic sea salt, which is high in magnesium and contains over 80 essential trace minerals)! Other natural foods high in good, usable sodium are: celery, kale, dandelion greens, spinach, and sea vegetables (such as laver, kelp, alaria and dulse).

Greens

The importance of eating mineral-rich green-leafy vegetables cannot be overstated. There are many greens to choose from (salad greens, lettuces, kale, chard, spinach, endive, etc.); find the ones you really enjoy and include them in your diet every day.

Green-leafy vegetables should be a powerhouse staple of any health-seeker's diet, and bodybuilders and those wanting to gain strength and muscle are no exception. Rid your mind of the idea that salad is "rabbit food" or "diet food."

Traveling

When traveling (or living) in third-world countries or other places where vegetable cleanliness is questionable, I highly recommend taking your mineral supplements with you. You will be glad you did!

*   *   *   *   *

It is interesting to note that of the 50,000 edible plant species in the world, just 15 crop plants provide over 90% of the foods the citizens of the world eat. And three of them, rice, corn and wheat, make up two thirds of this. It's no secret that the modern foods most deficient in minerals are...you guessed it, rice, corn and wheat. Again, a diet high in raw, organic, alkaline minerals is the goal. Don't do what the masses are doing. The herd is plundering into the abyss. Live like no one else so you can live like no one else.

Balance minerals, foods, and food classes to achieve specific physical, mental, emotional, and spiritual states.

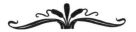

Absorption, Assimilation, and Digestion

It's not only what you eat,
it's what you absorb that counts.
— Dr. Bernard Jensen

If you are having trouble making weight and strength gains, you may have absorption, assimilation, and/or digestion problems. Have you ever known someone (maybe even yourself) who is very thin but eats large quantities of food? The reason for this phenomenon may be that the person is absorbing very little nutrients due to a layer of "plaque" on his or her intestinal tract. The intestinal villi cannot freely pull in nutrients. This layer inhibits crucial in and outflows of gastric and intestinal fluids. When these flows are hindered, the natural balance is offset, causing a chain reaction of nasty problems such as: a vitamin B-12 deficiency, diverticulitis, candida, leaky bowel syndrome, colitis, cysts and tumors.

The process of perfect absorption, assimilation, digestion, and elimination is the great secret of life. The better your absorption, assimilation, and digestion, the less you need to eat.

Another essential word of advice is to chew foods very well and eat slowly. Fletcherize your food. Dr. Fletcher taught that each mouthful of food should be chewed at least 50 times before swallowing. An ancient Indian proverb states: "Chew your food well, for the stomach has no teeth." Thoroughly mix the food with your saliva. The more your food is ground up and chewed, the greater the absorption by the body.

Often, the Standard American Diet cooked-food eater's intestinal tract is lined with a mucus layer which prevents nutriments from passing through the intestinal villi. This mucus must be broken up and dissolved to restore the proper functioning of the intestinal tract. I recommend a series of colon irrigations to jump-start the cleansing process for those who aren't able to do so through diet alone. Also, there are certain foods which efficiently dissolve mucus, such as the fig. The fig is ranked as one of the highest mucus dissolvers in Ragnar Berg's Table in Arnold Ehret's book Mucusless Diet Healing System.

Of course, raw-plant foods improve the total inner environment. Raw food greatly enhances the efficiency of nutrient absorption. Over time, a raw-food diet enables the body to dislodge and remove accumulated wastes from the intestinal folds. (Thor's Hammer tablets are a tremendous help to get digestion back on track. If you're green inside, you're clean inside.)

For mild cases of poor absorption, assimilation, and/or digestion, I recommend occasionally eating the cassia fruit. Cassia is the pod-fruit of a tree that is found in tropical regions. Cassia is a natural laxative which can play a crucial role in the early stages of a raw-food diet in order to facilitate the detoxification processes and to help alleviate constipation. Cassia discs are contained within the pod of the fruit. Each disc tastes like a cross between chocolate and carob and can be sucked on until it dissolves. Five to six discs should be enough to help with bowel movements. Each pod contains 40 plus discs.

For more severe cases of poor absorption, assimilation, and/or digestion, I highly recommend the Ejuva Body Cleansing Program. Having debated these issues for many years and worked with thousands of people, I highly recommend this herbal-intestinal cleanse program for anyone who experiences absorption, assimilation, and/or digestion problems. This is a 4-6 week herbal program involving increasing the intake of herbs and juices and decreasing the intake of food. Certain herbs contain compounds (especially when eaten in conjunction with one another) which force the digestive system to release mucoid plaque (encrusted mucus created by a lifetime of eating cooked foods, animal foods, medicine, etc.). These herbs are more effective in removing intestinal plaque than any green-leafy vegetable, fruit, or juice combination we have found. It is common to see mucoid plaque come out of people who have been eating 100% raw foods for over 3 years. Mucoid plaque is very difficult to relieve unless one is doing raw foods, juices and herbs. The Ejuva cleanse is 100% raw, 100% organic or wild, contains no fillers, no isolated compounds, no bentonite (bentonite has been shown to contain 22% aluminum), is 100% naturally dried, cut, sifted, and compressed into three different tablet formulations to be chewed up like food. Also included in the cleanse program are: a psyllium/flax/chia seed mix for juices while on the cleanse and a probiotic formulation. Simple, detailed instructions on how to follow the cleanse are included. This herbal intestinal rebuilding kit is a little pricey, but worth every penny (note: it is on sale at Rawpower.com every day).

Vitamin B-12 Deficiency

A vitamin B-12 deficiency can arise when there is a complete disruption in the human body's intestinal flora. In a normal situation vitamin B-12 is absorbed from bacteria in the intestinal tract. Most meat eaters are not afflicted by this deficiency because animal flesh (including insect tissue) contains a plethora of B-12. Maintaining adequate B12 levels on a raw-food vegan diet long term can be done by consuming Raw B-12, Vita Synergy multivitamin, Vitamineral Green, sea vegetables, AFA blue-green algae, spirulina and home-grown, freshly-picked, unwashed food (which provides the intestines with soil-based organisms which are transmutated in good intestinal flora which help create excellent B12 levels).

Additionally, excessive amounts of sweet fruit in the diet can cause the intestinal flora to become sterilized (sugar is an antibiotic). Eat more greens, algaes, and drink more green juices. Get out in the sun daily.

Lastly, be cautioned that chlorinated tap water can sterilize the intestinal flora as well.

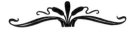

Exercise and Weight Training

A lot of us are busy with work, family and so many commitments. The workout time can be viewed as the one hour of the day you dedicate to yourself.

Muscles provide the ground-work for genuine physical beauty. A healthy physique can be developed by muscular development, sunshine on the skin, deep-breathing, and proper control of weight by eating naturally and sensibly. Both men and women can build beautiful sculpted muscles through intense resistance exercise. Remember, 50% of the body's weight is muscle.

Total fitness has three vital components: aerobic conditioning, flexibility, and muscular conditioning.

Aerobic activity is anything that uses up a lot of oxygen. Oxygen is delivered to the muscles by the cardiovascular system—the lungs, heart, and circulation of the blood. The system is developed by continuous, high-repetition exercise such as running, swimming, jumping rope, riding a bicycle, etc.

Muscles, tendons, and ligaments tend to shorten over a period of time, which limits our range of motion and renders us more vulnerable to injury when sudden stresses are placed on these body parts. But we can counteract this tendency by stretching exercises and stretching programs.

The best way to develop and strengthen the muscles is

resistance training. When you contract the muscles against resistance, they adapt to this level of effort. The best and most efficient way of doing this is through weight training.

To gain strength and muscular weight, do progressive, anaerobic exercise six days a week, giving yourself one day off. Push yourself—be physical! And think *powerfully*. Remember, the Mind is the most important factor.

Do the exercises you feel good doing—those which agree with you. You can exercise anywhere. Exercise whenever you watch television, listen to the radio or audio books, etc., but be on guard against the negative, hypnotic suggestion of mass media. Keep in mind that participating in mass media contributes to a negative attitude and a negative outlook on life, so avoid it whenever possible. (When we were teenagers, my brother and I used to pass a dumbbell back and forth while we watched a movie or sporting event, doing sets of exercises until whatever we were watching was over.)

To gain healthy weight and build muscular size or strength, you must perform exercise feats which you are not presently capable of doing. You must attempt the momentarily impossible. This is what separates success from failure.

Do exercises which are difficult yet safe, which you enjoy, and which suit your lifestyle. Preferably, exercise outdoors under the sun or, in the alternative, at a home-gym or convenient facility. Exercise at a convenient time of day or night, as frequently as possible, and as regularly as possible. Choose a program you will follow throughout your life.

Start your exercise program with amounts of weight and repetitions which are easy to perform. Advance gradually and increase slowly. Muscles should be contracted to their fullest extent and joints should be carried through their full range of movement. Place demands on your body within reasonable limits. Once the muscles are warmed up, then conduct short periods of intense, vigorous, extremely resistant exercise. This will put more muscle weight on your body than maintaining a long period of mild exercise.

To gain weight, do more anaerobic (without oxygen) exercises than aerobic (with oxygen) exercises in your workout. Aerobic exercise is good for your heart and helps you gain endurance, not muscular development.

Examples of aerobic exercises are: walking, jogging, long-distance running, dancing, long-distance swimming, long-distance cycling, cross-country skiing, etc.

To gain weight and develop muscles, do anaerobic exercises. Anaerobic exercises are heavy exercises such as: lifting heavy weights, sprinting, wrestling, rope climbing, jumping, speed cycling, sprint swimming, etc.

A fantastic exercise is swimming underwater, or doing underwater laps in a pool. Swimming is an aerobic activity, but when you swim underwater while holding your breath, you greatly increase your lung capacity, which will help your weightlifting workout. You will see a big difference in your breathing after a few weeks of doing the exercise consistently.

Anaerobic exercises are intense exercises which can only be tolerated for a few moments. They are short bursts of high-energy activities. They use muscle groups at high intensities which exceed the body's capacity to use oxygen to supply energy. They create an oxygen debt by using energy produced without oxygen. They are activities which demand such a great mus-

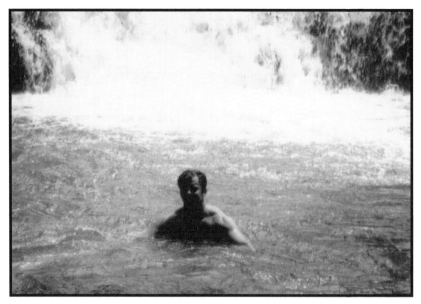

I recommend doing laps under water while holding your breath. Also, treading water for 30 minutes after an intense work-out really gives your body an extra boost and gives you an edge over everyone else!

cle explosion that the body has to rely upon an internal metabolic process for oxygen.

Breathe between anaerobic exertions. Take deep, diaphragmatic breaths. Anaerobic exercises may be: isotonic, isokinetic, isometric, and/or negative or "eccentric" exercises.

Isotonic exercise involves movement of a constant heavy weight through a full range of possible movement. It is a muscular action in which there is a change in the length of the muscle, while the tension remains constant. The bench press is a classic example of an isotonic exercise.

Isokinetic exercise is exercise in which there is accommodation resistance and constant speed. Nautilus is a type of isokinetic machine where the machine varies the amount of resistance being lifted to match the force curve developed by the muscle. Isokinetics is exercising in which the maximum force of which the muscle is capable of is applied throughout the range of motion.

Isometric exercise involves a static contraction. It is the application of a high percentage of your existing strength against an unmoving resistance, a fixed limit. Isometrics entails pushing against an immovable force such as: another set of opposing muscles, a wall, building, door, bar, taught rope, towel, two-ton truck, etc. If you push hard enough, you feel stress on your muscles. In isometrics, each exercise should be practiced at several joint angles. Training at many angles distributes the strength gains throughout the range of the muscle's movement. In isometrics, each "all-out" push or pull should be held as long as possible, to the point of muscular failure. Isometric exercises can be done practically anywhere. They are simple and effective. Isometrics increase the strength and improve the muscles' tone and shape. Isometric exercise entails muscular contraction where the muscle maintains a constant length and the joints do not move.

In negative or "eccentric" exercises, you lower the weight very slowly, at a smooth, steady pace, without interrupting the downward movement. In positive or "concentric" exercise, you raise the weight at normal speed. In negative exercise, your muscle is stretching and lengthening while maintaining tension against resistance. In positive exercise, the muscle is contracting and shortening against resistance. In negative exercise, you resist pressure and in positive exercise, you apply pressure. The muscle has the ability to handle more force during negative exercise than it can during positive exercise. For example, when performing a bench press, the positive part of the repetition is the portion during which the weight is being pressed from the chest to arm's length. The negative portion of the repetition is the part during which the weight is lowered back down to the chest. In negative pull-ups, you climb into the top position using your legs, so that you simply lower yourself back down. Negative parallel bar dips can be done in the same way.

All four of these anaerobic exercise types, isotonic, isokinetic, isometric, and/or negative or "eccentric," should be employed as part of your workout program.

My personal exercise program is one that combines weight-training and yogic principles. These principles include: focused, intentional breathing, prolonged muscular contractions, correct posture and alignment, and deep relaxation.

A Word About Sex

Boxers, horse trainers, and successful athletes have long understood that abstinence from sex before a competition maintains strength. Overindulgence in sex, with the resultant loss of nutrients during ejaculation, causes weight loss and energy depletion. After ejaculation, nutrients designed for other vital organs are sidetracked into the production of reproductive materials. This depletion results in a momentary insufficiency in the nutrients available to other biological systems of the body. Sex is wonderful, but engage in sex at the appropriate times—not before a workout or contest!

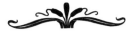

Sunshine

Separation from sunlight will result in disease, just as surely as will separation from fresh air, food, and water.
— Dr. Zane Kime

The human organism is solar-powered. All life on this spinning planet is sustained directly or indirectly by the sun. If you want to build muscle and strength, it is important to get adequate sunshine. Healthy doses of sunlight quicken the detoxification process and lay a solid foundation for healing and muscle building.

A common myth is that the sun "causes" skin cancer. Humans have thrived under the sun for millions of years. Only in the last 70 years or so has the incidence of skin cancer dramatically increased. What else has happened in that time frame? The industrialization of food. In other words, that is when denatured and highly processed foods entered the Standard American Diet—in a big way.

The field of science is now looking into the link between diet and skin cancer. The kinds of fats (polyunsaturated) and the amounts (way too much!) people living in industrialized nations eat, and the lack of rich antioxidant foods in their diets (read: not enough raw fruits and vegetables!) are proving to be directly linked to skin cancer.

It is estimated by experts that at least 70% of Americans

are deficient in vitamin D. This deficiency is one of the root causes of many dangerous chronic diseases (including cancer, diabetes, and heart disease). Since vitamin D is created under the skin by ultraviolet light, we need to be exposed to sunshine or use supplements. (There is one vitamin D product I recommend to people who live in a cold climate with periods of no direct sunlight, called RAW D3, but a healthy amount of sunshine on the skin is the best choice.)

Get outside for exercise every day you can. You cannot gain strength and healthy weight if you are sitting indoors all day. The best place to exercise is not in an artificial, air-conditioned gym, but in the green outdoors among the living plants, wild animals, and fresh air. If you want to lift heavy weights, bring them outside and exercise in the open air with the sky above. If you feel you can do without them, do not wear shoes, gloves, or belts. Lift weights with as little clothing on as possible. "Gymnasium" means "to train in the nude." (However, always keep in mind your own safety when engaged in these activities, of course.)

Sunlight and fresh air aid the metobolic and healing processes of the body. You will never feel better than when your body is in shape and you have a good color to your skin. Thinness is associated with paleness. I have also found that people who are afraid of fruit are usually afraid of the sun and afraid of exercise. So, eat fruit, get out in the sun, and exercise!

It you live where skies are often overcast, or winters are cold and long, it is still important to get outside every day you can. Some sunlight can almost always get through cloud cover and a little bit of sunshine on your face and arms every day will make a big difference. When the body is warmed up by the sun, the tissues expand. Thus, you may find in the summer it is easier to gain strength and weight under the warm summer sun.

Don't buy into the demonization of sunshine! You just need internal protection from the sun's rays in the form of proper, natural, raw-food nutrition, and the common sense to know when to retreat to shade to discontinue sun exposure.

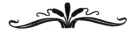

Hydration

I drink six or seven glasses of water a day.
I also drink fresh vegetable juice.
And I have at least five or six pieces of
fresh fruit every day, and ten raw vegetables.
— Jack LaLanne

It is well known that people who have more muscle need more water. Muscles are comprised of about 70% water (the same percentage of the earth's surface) and they need to stay hydrated to function properly. Dehydration is actually the precursor to the cause of countless ailments. Even mild dehydration can tire you out prematurely and weaken your muscles.

How much water should we drink in order to stay hydrated? Experts have determined that, for normal hydration, you should divide your body weight in pounds by two and drink that many ounces of water each day. I've heard that more active, muscular people should be drinking even more than that. With our busy lives, it can be difficult to remember to drink this much water every day, so what I do is drink 24 ounces first thing in the morning, then every time I urinate during the day, I'll immediately drink 8-10 ounces of water, then before bed, I'll drink another 12-16 ounces. This system works well for me.

Most of the time when people think they're hungry, they're actually dehydrated (thirsty). An important thing to remember is to not wait until you're thirsty to drink water—by then, it's too late and you are already somewhat dehydrated.

Our bodies use up a lot of water every day. Most is excreted through the skin (sweat) and kidneys (urine) and with each exhalation of breath (just breathe onto a mirror). Yes, even the simple act of breathing causes us to use about 16 ounces of water each day.

Because water helps with our digestion, elimination and metabolism, people gain bodyfat when they don't drink enough water. Water is vital to every aspect of your body's physiological function.

Always drink filtered, purified, distilled or clean spring water (know the spring source), and from a glass or stainless steel container, not plastic (especially not dark plastic). Plastic leaches toxins into your water and into you.

Also, I recommend that everyone uses a whole-house water filtration system, especially if municipal city water flows into your home. We all know how polluted tap water is and if you're bathing in it, your skin is absorbing all the waterborne toxins and heavy metals in it. As I've said for years, "Use a water filter, or you will become one!"

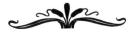

Sleep, Rest and Meditation

Protest the war that's being waged inside your mind.

Getting enough sleep is vitally important to building strength and muscle mass. Sleep plays a major role in protein synthesis, the release of growth hormones, and, of course, reenergizes you for the upcoming day. Sleep gives you more energy than any food can. Probably the most important part of the recovery cycle is getting adequate sleep. In fact, up to 90% of muscle growth occurs during sleep!

Try to grab a short nap (20 minutes) sometime after your post-workout smoothie or meal. Most people can't squeeze it into their day, but the ones who can know how powerful and helpful to muscle recovery and growth it is. Just sitting quietly and clearing your mind once or twice a day is also very helpful.

Have you ever known someone who could not, to put it bluntly, just shut up for 60 seconds? Someone who just could not sit still? Someone who needed constant outside stimulation? When I was younger, I knew a girl who could not close her eyes for 60 seconds. She could not sit still for 30 seconds. And she could not keep her mouth shut for 10 seconds! She was truly the stereotypical "chicken with its head cut off." As amusing as this sounds, it is extremely detrimental to one's health to not be able to sit calmly with one's eyes closed and mouth shut, thus emptying one's mind of "chatter."

Meditation is not an obscure Indian method, it is not simply a technique, it is a way of being. Meditation is the greatest adventure the human mind can undertake. It is when you are not doing anything at all. Meditation is a state in which your mind is completely void of any thought, your body completely void of any movement, and your persona void of any emotion.

This emptying of the mind is wonderful and liberating. It is invigorating and it prepares you to re-enter the world fresh and focused. I have found it to be an essential part of my bodybuilding program. One's mind must be clear and focused to perform potentially dangerous feats of strength.

The best book I've come across on this subject is entitled Meditation: The First and Last Freedom by Osho. It is a practical guide for one who desires to quiet the chatter of the mind and achieve self-mastery. I have been recommending this book to people for years.

Also, a really cool thing to try if you are adventurous is a meditation session in a floatation tank. In my opinion, floating (as it's called) is the doorway to profound relaxation and altered states. Your mind and body can experience a sensory overload from daily life and a floatation tank can help you maintain your equilibrium by freeing your mind and body. Basically, what happens is the odorless tank is void of light and sound, so your smell, sight, and hearing senses are relieved. The tank's water is filled with hundreds of pounds of Epsom salt to make you 100% buoyant. This will relieve you of your sense of gravity and, in turn, will begin the process of reversing the harmful effects of gravity. The water is heated to your exact body temperature, relieving you of all sense of temperature. You are in the tank for an hour or so. You enter into a different realm of being. I've done it a few times and it is an amazing experience. I came out of there a new person, no doubt about it.

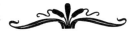

Raw Bodybuilding Foods

Following is a list of raw foods I have used over the years to help build strength and muscle. Some of these foods can be found at your local natural food co-op or health-food store. Others are foods I have sourced for my own use over the years and now distribute at Rawpower.com.

Part I
Raw Bodybuilding Foods Available from
Your Local Food Co-op or Health-Food Store

Greens, Greens, Greens

As stated earlier in this book, green-leafy vegetables are some of the most important foods for anyone interested in health and fitness, and are of great importance to those wishing to gain strength and muscle. I can't say enough about what building foods green-leafy vegetables are, so I'll just let them speak for themselves: lettuce greens, dandelion greens, kale, chard, watercress (and all the cresses—winter cress, nasturtium, land cress, etc.), spinach, collard greens, arugula, endive, parsley, cilantro, romaine, mustard greens, sorrels... Don't be afraid of greens; be adventurous and enjoy trying new greens; find out which greens you like the most and include them in your daily diet.

Celery

Celery is one of the most nutritious foods known and is an important building food. Jay Kordich, The Juiceman, calls celery the "powerhouse of life-giving nutrition." Celery is high in water, so it replaces valuable fluids lost in sweat. Celery/apple juice has the perfect sodium-potassium ratio (1:5) which is all-important to prevent and relieve muscle cramping and fatigue (see recipe for Post Running or Hiking Drink in the Recipes section of this book).

Cabbage

Cabbage is often overlooked as it is not dark green and many people have memories of the putrid smell of cooked cabbage. Cabbage has sometimes been called the king of the cruciferous family. It is highly alkalinizing, cleansing, and rejuvenating and contains substantial amounts of sulfur, iodine, iron, vitamins C and E and is loaded with the amino acid glutamine. It also happens to be one of the least expensive vegetables (see recipe for Cabbage Wraps in the recipe section of this book).

Coconuts

If young coconuts are not available at your food co-op or natural food store, check the Asian markets near you. These are the young, fresh coconuts and are white on the outside. The brown hairy things you see are usually old and dry.

Grains

Even though they are traditionally thought of as starchy foods, some grains can add a substantial amount of protein to one's diet when they are sprouted. As opposed to the breakdown of cooked grains, the complex carbohydrates in sprouted grains, along with their available protein, break down into simpler sugars and readily absorbed amino acids. Whole grains are also a source of vegetable lignans, those great anti-cancer, hormone balancing, health-promoting phytochemicals. Jack LaLanne said,

"It's important to add grains to your diet because grains contain some nutrients that are not found in fruits and vegetables."

Part II
Raw Bodybuilding Foods
Available from Rawpower.com

Raw Olives

What if there was something that was 100% natural that would increase your strength and give you instant and blazing energy to get through your workouts? One of the best raw body-building foods is the olive. When I first discovered raw olives, I referred to them as "my Dianabol." Who needs steroids when raw olives are available? Olives are also the number one mucus-dissolving fruit and the fruit highest in minerals.

To be clear, I am not talking about the shiny, black (dyed), canned olives at the supermarket, nor the oily, lye-cured, olives in the "gourmet" olive bar, nor unripe, green, pickled olives. I am referring to ripe olives that have been sun dried/cured and ripe olives that have been cured in sea salt and water. The best raw olives I have found are:

Kalamata-Style Olives (aka Raw Power! Olives) — These delicious raw, sustainably-grown reddish-brown olives are packed in pure water with fresh garlic, a dash of fresh oregano, one ripe cayenne pepper, and Celtic sea salt. (These have been my favorite olives for over a decade—great atop a green salad or just eaten alone.)

Sun-Ripened Black Olives — These are raw, organic, sun-ripened olives, without any dyes to make them black. Prepared four ways: Plain and Unsalted, Herbed, Spiced, and Botija Olives in sea salt brine. I enjoy all four of these fabulous, moist olives.

Stone-Crushed Olive Oil

Olive oil is also quite powerful and is an essential in the raw, living-foods kitchen. The best olive oil I have found is Bariani stone-crushed olive oil. This olive oil is made from ripe olives that are crushed and ground with stone presses using the original techniques developed by the Greeks and Romans thousands of years ago. This oil is true to the original varieties available in the Mediterranean.

Raw Organic Nuts

Nuts are high in minerals and fat, both crucial to muscle building and overall health. Nuts also give you a grounded and full feeling. Nuts that I enjoy are macadamias, almonds, cashews, hazelnuts, pistachios, walnuts, and pecans. Cashews are the nut of choice for most raw-food chefs. Note: try to only buy nuts from businesses located in colder areas. Storing nuts in warm places can make them go rancid much more quickly.

Nut and Seed Butters

Raw, organic, almond butter is a treat few can resist. It is a very heavy, powerful food. It is also considered a "convenience food" by raw-foodists. I know a guy who is in sales and he travels all over. He always has a jar of almond butter and a spoon in his car. If he ever gets stuck in traffic or is far from home or another food source, he just digs into his almond butter! My wife usually makes her nut milks from "scratch," but when she's pressed for time, she makes nut milk from almond butter. She uses one half of a jar of almond butter (about 3/4 C), 1-5 large pitted dates, and 3-4 cups of water. She blends them all in the Vita-Mix and has almost instant nut milk! Pumpkin seed butter is one of the most delicious and nutritious treats you will ever taste. It tastes like peanut butter, but is much healthier.

Coconut Oil

Raw coconut oil (or coconut butter) is an instant energy source, contains no cholesterol (and has actually been found to lower cholesterol), no trans-fatty acids, and is not hydrogenated. Contrary to commercial oil industry propaganda, unprocessed coconut oil is a very good dietary fat source. Coconut oil is actually lower in calories than most other oils and a little goes a long way. It is also great for use as a skin moisturizer.

Seeds

Like nuts, seeds are mineral rich and high in fat and are filling and satisfying. Pumpkin seeds are one of the most important seeds for muscle building. In addition to having many other health benefits, they contain myosin, the main protein that makes up almost all the muscles in the body and plays an important role in muscular contraction. With their high magnesium, zinc and omega-3 fatty acid content, pumpkin seeds are a most helpful food for supporting male prostate health. Hemp seeds are high in complete protein, bountiful in essential fatty acids, and they taste great (something like a cross between sesame seeds and peanuts.) Chia seeds are also very nutritional. "Chia," the Mayan word for "Strength," is a complete protein, providing all of the amino acids necessary to support even the most active lifestyle. Its abundant water soluble fiber may lower cholesterol and regulate blood sugar. As one of the plant kingdom's richest sources of omega 3 and 6 essential fatty acids, it supports strong nails, lustrous hair, and a glowing complexion.

Most everyone interested in health and nutrition is now familiar with the health benefits of flax seeds. Rich in essential fatty acids, dietary fiber and lignans, flax seeds have been found to protect heart and artery functions, build the immune system, soothe intestinal problems, relieve constipation, aid in detoxification, balance estrogen levels (comparable to soy), reduce arthritis and other inflammation... the list goes on and on. Raw Power carries a variety of raw, organic flax crackers and snacks.

Sun-Dried Fruit

Sun-dried fruit is high in minerals and energizing fruit sugars. My favorite sun-dried fruit, apricots, are especially high in magnesium (known as the "anabolic" mineral) and potassium, minerals that supply us with energy, stamina, and endurance. They contain iron for blood building and silicon for healthy skin and hair.

Dried Berries

Berries are high in vitamins and minerals and they taste great. Bears eat large amounts of berries as part of their diet and they gain massive weight and strength from doing so. One type of berries called goji berries are perhaps the most nutritionally dense fruit known. They contain 18 kinds of amino acids (six times higher than bee pollen) and contain all eight essential amino acids. Goji berries contain up to 21 trace minerals and are one of the richest sources of carotenoids of all known foods on earth! When ground into a fine, raw powder, they contain hundreds of times more vitamin C, by weight, than oranges, making them second only to camu camu berries as the richest vitamin C source. They are also high in vitamins B-1, B-2, B-6, and E. Goji berries contain polysaccharides which fortify the immune system. One polysaccharide found in this fruit has been found to be a powerful secretagogue (a substance that stimulates the secretion of rejuvenative human growth hormone by the pituitary gland). Goji berries have been traditionally regarded as a longevity, strength-building, and sexual potency food of the highest order.

Sea Vegetables

The health benefits of sea vegetables are numerous. They are loaded with minerals and trace elements and are a great source of healthful sodium. A few of my favorites are:

Dulse — Dulse is a red seaweed with flat, fan-shaped fronds that grows from the temperate to frigid zones of the Atlantic and Pacific. Dulse makes a great addition to salads. This alkaline vegetable is an excellent source of iron and many trace minerals. It also contains iodine and manganese, which activate enzyme systems.

Laver (Nori) — Nori (also called Laver) is a dark red, lavender seaweed. It can be added to salads or is great to snack on as-is. Nori has the highest protein contents of any seaweed (48% of dry weight). It also contains an enzyme that helps break down cholesterol deposits. Nori is high in vitamins A, B-1, B-3 (niacin), and trace minerals.

Nori Sheets — This raw, sun-dried nori has been processed into thin sheets which can be used to make nori rolls and other raw-food meals and treats.

Bee Pollen

Bee pollen is the pollen produced by flowers that honey bees gather and bring back to the hive. Pollen grains are microscopic in size and bees collect millions of these individual grains and connect them with nectar into small pellets. Conscious bee-keepers use a collection device that harvests a small percentage of the bee pollen pellets as the bees return to the hive. The bees are never harmed, and sufficient pollen gets through to provide for the hive's needs. Bee pollen is an alkaline food considered by many nutritionists to be the most complete food found in nature.

It is a rich source of high-quality protein and contains all essential amino acids and an abundance of minerals, making it a great strength-builder and brain food. Some of the benefits of bee pollen consumption include: increased energy and stamina, increased muscle growth and definition, immune system fortification, antioxidant activity, enhanced sexuality, and smoothed wrinkles.

Raw Food Energy Bars

Energy bars are here to stay—they are valued fuel foods for those who are active, athletic, on-the-go, and busy but want to eat nutritiously when away from home or after work-outs. Thankfully, there are now some great raw-food bars available.

At Rawpower.com, we carry several high-quality raw, organic bars and everyone has their favorite. My favorites are the Raw Crunch Bars (Blueberry and Goji Berry). These are the raw-foodist's solution to protein and energy bars. They're so much better tasting and much better for you than those supermarket bars with the *long* lists of ingredients! Raw Crunch Bars are made from raw, organic ingredients, minimally-processed, great-tasting, high in fiber and made without additives. Plus, they are hand made by Kathy Feldman Leveque, National Fitness Competitor and author of The Raw Crunch Diet. Invest in a case of these bars and watch your energy skyrocket during your work-outs.

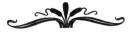

Superfoods

*Some people don't "believe" in superfoods.
It doesn't have anything to do with belief—it is a <u>fact</u>
that some foods are vastly superior to others in terms
of purity, density of nutrients, degree of mineralization, etc.*

A superfood is a food which contains unique (and even medicinal), health-promoting properties. These are foods which are more nutrient-rich, or concentrated, than normal foods and typically have higher levels of vitamins, minerals, antioxidants, amino acids, etc. than commonly-consumed foods. Superfoods allow us to eat less, but take in more nutrients at the same time. As I mentioned earlier in the book, you want to be eating the most unharmful, most nutrient-rich foods possible. This is what eating superfoods is all about. After 15 years of eating raw foods and trying different approaches, my conclusion is that the best diet is one in which a combination of fresh raw foods and concentrated dried superfoods are eaten.

Following, I list some of my favorite superfoods. Optimally, all superfoods should be organically grown and eaten in their raw (uncooked) state. I use these superfoods as ingredients, or "boosts," in my Raw Power Smoothies, salads, recipes, trail mixes, etc. (See Raw Power Recipes chapter for numerous smoothie ideas.)

Berries

In my opinion, berries are the best foods on Earth. I eat as many berries as I can, every chance I get. In the summer, our family gorges on several varieties of berries we get at the local organic farmers' market, and we go hiking to forage for thimbleberries, which (along with huckleberries) grow abundantly in the wild where we live in Northern Idaho. Search out which berries grow wildly near where you live, and get them before the critters do!

Goji Berries — Rarely do you have a fruit that packs this much nutrition into such a delicious little package. With their impressive combination of protein and beneficial nutrients, it's no wonder these tasty little berries have become the world's most popular superfood. Nutritionally, goji berries are an amazing source of vitamin C, beta carotene, polysaccharides, amino acids, zinc, copper, and many other nutrients. According to Traditional Chinese Medicine practitioners, goji berries are also considered quite beneficial in helping to bring more chi into the body. Always seek raw, sundried, certified organic goji berries as there are hundreds of cheap, pesticide-ridden versions out there on the market today. Goji Berry Extract Powder is also a great addition to any super smoothie.

Blueberries have a diverse range of nutrients, with notably high levels of the essential dietary mineral manganese, vitamin B-6, vitamin C, vitamin K and dietary fiber. Blueberries contain anthocyanins, other antioxidant pigments and various phytochemicals having a role in reducing risks of diseases, including inflammation and certain cancers. This all-around, amazing superfood has been shown to enhance memory and stimulate brain activity. Blueberries can be distinguished from the nearly identical looking bilberries by cutting them in half. Ripe blueberries have white or light green flesh, while bilberries and huckleberries are red or purple throughout. Bilberries are most often found singularly or in pairs, while blueberries are most often found in clusters.

Commonly confused with blueberries, bilberries are recognized as a good source of flavonoids which have strong antioxidative activity. The fruit is smaller than that of the blueberry but with a fuller taste. As a deep purple fruit, bilberries contain anthocyanin pigments. In folk medicine, bilberry leaves were used to treat gastrointestinal ailments, applied topically, or made into infusions. Bilberries are known to improve eyesight and also used as a tonic to prevent some infections and skin diseases. Bilberries are softer and juicier than blueberries, making them difficult to transport. If you can find fresh, ripe bilberries, don't pass them up!

The state fruit of Idaho, huckleberries, are a great source of vitamin C and antioxidants. Although similar in appearance, huckleberries have a noticeable, distinct taste different from blueberries and are enjoyed by many mammals, including grizzly bears and humans. I enjoy adding fresh, wild huckleberries to my summer smoothies.

Acai Berries are high in dietary fiber, rich in antioxidants, healthy fatty acids, vitamin A and calcium. Many value acai for increased energy, healthier skin, and an immune system boost. Mixing acai powder into drinks or smoothies is a great way to add ooomph and nutrition to your diet. Acai powder contains 30 times more antioxidants than found in red wine, and almost always finds its way into my daily super smoothies.

Red raspberries contain significant amounts of antioxidants such as anthocyanin pigments. Raspberries are a rich source of vitamin C, manganese and dietary fiber. In fact, they are among the foods with the highest fiber content known, up to

20% fiber per total weight. Ranking near the top of all fruits antioxidant content, raspberries have an ORAC value (oxygen radical absorbance capacity) of about 4900 per 100 grams, making them among the top-ranked ORAC fruits.

Camu Camu Berries — Harvested by hand from the banks of the Amazon, this incredible superfruit is the highest natural source of vitamin C—with hundreds of times more than oranges when dried into a raw powder! Unlike synthetic vitamin supplements, Camu Camu contains all the vital flavonoids and co-factors that synergize together in your body. Camu Camu powder is intense. Add just a teaspoon to smoothies and juices for a super-nutrient boost, especially during cold and flu season!

Blackberries (no, not the cell phones!) are very seedy and not the most fun berry to eat, however they are a very good source of dietary fiber, vitamin C, vitamin K and manganese. Because they are so seedy, I find them a great choice to blend into my morning smoothies.

If you've never tried goldenberries (also called Incan Berries) before, you're in for quite a treat. Popular in Europe as a chocolate-covered delicacy, these tart, tangy snacks are an amazing source of vitamin C, flavonoids, and protein, to name just a few of their nutritional benefits. Goldenberries are delicious right out of the bag and are great in trail mixes, desserts, and a wide variety of other recipes.

Mulberries are a good source of dietary fiber, riboflavin, magnesium and potassium, and a very good source of vitamin C, vitamin K and iron. Mulberries are also a good source of resveratrol, a potent phytonutrient also found in grapes that researchers believe can prevent cancer and aid in the fight of existing cancers. They are also low in sodium, and very low in saturated fat and cholesterol. In Traditional Chinese Medicine, mulberries are considered a blood tonic (meaning that they cleanse the blood and increase its production, strengthening the entire system), are believed to strengthen the kidneys, to be effective in cleansing the liver, and to strengthen one's hearing and vision. Folk lore has it that mulberries help prevent premature graying of the hair. Modern nutritionists wonder if there isn't a kernel of truth in that lore having to do with the high mineral profile of mulberries.

Traditionally used medicinally for hundreds of years, elderberries are used for their high antioxidant activity, to lower cholesterol, to improve vision, to boost the immune system, to improve heart health and for coughs, colds, flu, bacterial and viral infections and tonsilitis. Bioflavonoids and other proteins in elderberries destroy the ability of cold and flu viruses to infect a cell.

Amla berries have been used to treat various diseases through Ayurvedic medicine therapy dating back many centuries. They contain a high concentration of vitamin C and potent antioxidants. Amla is also popularly used in shampoos and hair oil treatments.

Again, eat as many berries as you can get your hands on!

Vegetables and Greens

Celery is commonly used in weight-loss diets because it provides low-calorie dietary fiber. However, celery is one of the main bodybuilding vegetables because of its high natural sodium content. It's also a very good source of vitamin A, vitamin C, vitamin K, folate, potassium and manganese. Celery can be thought of as a "free" food—meaning you can eat as much of it as you want, whenever you want.

Purple (red) cabbage is a great food, especially as part of

a post-workout meal as it is high in glutamine, an amino acid that plays an important role in protein synthesis, muscle growth and nitrogen donation for many anabolic processes. This nutrient-packed and low-calorie food contains high levels of calcium, iron, iodine, potassium, sulfur, and phosphorus and is loaded with vitamins A, B-1, B-2, B-6, C, E, K and folic acid. Study after study has shown that fresh cabbage juice has been effective in the treatment of a number of cancers and ulceration in the digestive tracts. In our home, no green salad or vegetable plate is complete without chopped or shredded purple cabbage. We also use the sturdy leaves as "shells" or "wraps" for our raw-food creations (see recipe for Cabbage Wraps in the recipe section of this book). This superfood is a daily staple for our family.

Even though fresh vegetable juices and green juices, are blends, or mixtures, I classify them as superfoods because they are so important to a person venturing into a raw-food diet. Not only do they help in keeping you hydrated, they are very nourishing and bodybuilding. You want to use a good quality juice extractor when you are making these health elixirs. Use a juicer that extracts not only the liquid, but the micronutrients, such as the trace minerals, as well. You also want to use one that leaves little waste when you are juicing. This will save you lots of money and lots of extra trips to the market over your lifetime. My family and I use the Green Star GS-2000 and we love it. It works perfectly and generates very little waste (pulp). The money you will save on produce over the years of using this juice extractor will more than pay for the cost of the juicer.

It is said that Incan warriors consumed maca root to increase strength and endurance. Modern health seekers look to maca when they need improved ability to deal with stress, increased energy, more endurance and better performance. Maca is rich in essential minerals (including calcium and iron). Maca's reported beneficial effects for sexual function could be due to its high concentration of proteins, fatty acids and vital nutrients. Blend maca into a smoothie for an energizing start to a healthy day.

Organic Purple Corn Extract Powder has just about the highest known antioxidant content of any food—even more than blueberries! Since ancient times, people have soaked purple corn kernels in water to make a purple drink called chicha. Today, the benefits of purple corn are available in this concentrated powder, to give your smoothies and energy drinks a purple-powered antioxidant kick. (My wife also likes that it lends a great color to some smoothies that would otherwise be brownish-orangish-greenish, and this can be helpful with kids.) Rich in beneficial phenolics and anthocyanins.

Barley Grass Powder provides a broad range of nutrients including healthy alkaline minerals, chlorophyll, fiber and phytonutrients. It has been said that while barley grass doesn't contain every necessary nutrient, it comes closer than just about any other food. It has been used in traditional Chinese medicine for over 1,800 years.

Wheatgrass juice is high in chlorophyll and has an abundance of phytochemicals, antioxidants and vitamin K. Other vitamins and nutrients include vitamin C, vitamin E, vitamin B-12, beta-carotene, phosphorus, magnesium, potassium, calcium, iron, folic acid, 90 different minerals and 20 amino acids (a complete protein). I consumed so much wheatgrass juice when I first adopted a raw-food diet that my raw food friends called me Captain Wheatgrass!

Romaine lettuce is my lettuce of choice. Unlike most lettuces, dark green romaine is more tolerant of warmer temperatures, so it stays crisp in transit (great when taking lunch to work, taking salads on picnics or to parties, etc.). As with other dark leafy greens, the antioxidants contained within romaine lettuce are believed to help prevent cancer. Perfect for salads, blending into a green smoothie, using as a "shell" or "wrap" for your raw-food meals, or munching on as-is. Other green and red lettuces are excellent as well: red leaf, green curly, butterhead, etc. Experiment and find your favorite lettuces.

Spinach has a high nutritional value and is extremely rich in antioxidants, especially when fresh. It is a rich source of vitamin A, vitamin C, vitamin E, vitamin K, magnesium, manganese, folate, betaine, iron, vitamin B-2, calcium, potassium, vitamin B-6, folic acid, copper, protein, phosphorus, zinc, niacin, selenium and omega-3 fatty acids. Turns out Popeye was right (although he consumed canned, cooked, commercial spinach!). Eat your spinach fresh, raw, organic and often!

Kale is a highly nutritious vegetable with powerful antioxidant properties and is considered to be anti-inflammatory. Kale is very high in beta carotene, vitamin K, vitamin C, lutein, zeaxanthin, and reasonably rich in calcium. Kale, as with broccoli and other brassicas, contains sulforaphane (particularly when chopped or minced), a chemical believed to have potent anti-cancer properties. Kale is also a good source of carotenoids. Fresh, raw, organic kale is a common ingredient in my freshly-made green juices. My wife also makes a fantastic marinated kale salad.

Cilantro is the fresh leafy part of the coriander plant. Its distinct taste livens up many raw-food meals and recipes and is a very good source of dietary fiber, vitamin A, vitamin C, vitamin E, vitamin K, riboflavin, niacin, vitamin B-6, folate, pantothenic acid, calcium, iron, magnesium, phosphorus, potassium, copper and manganese. Behind only chlorella, cilantro is the number two food that best assists the body in the detoxification of heavy metals.

Nuts

Brazil Nuts are a healthy, lower-cost alternative to almonds. Just two of them meet your daily requirement for the anti-cancer mineral selenium! Selenium is one of the most important minerals and also one of the minerals most people are deficient in, especially men. Brazil nuts contain heart-healthy mono-unsaturated oils and a full spectrum of amino acids. Brazil Nut Protein Powder is made by pressing the nuts, thus extracting out the oil (fat content). What's left is the protein-rich fiber. Added to smoothies, it provides plenty of protein, with a full spectrum of amino acids and hundreds of times more selenium than any other nut!

Raw cashews are prized for their versatility as much as their unique flavor. They can be used in smoothies, made into nut milk, used as a base for vegetable dips and salad dressings, blended with berries and dates into a simple but delicious pudding, etc. Of course, they are also perfect for eating as-is or adding to healthy homemade trail mixes. Most cashews labelled "raw" have been steamed at high temperatures to remove their shells. Raw Power Cashews have been shelled by hand, leaving the nut raw and with all of its beneficial enzymes intact.

Almonds are high in vitamin E and are rich in monounsaturated fat, one of the two "good" fats responsible for lowering LDL cholesterol. Great for snacking right out of the bag, adding to healthy, homemade trail mixes, or using in your favorite healthy recipes.

Walnuts are rich in fiber, B vitamins, magnesium, and antioxidants. They have significantly higher amounts of Omega 3 fatty acids than other nuts. Good for heart health and function, even the FDA has recognized the benefits of walnuts in heart disease prevention. Eat them instead of foods that are high in saturated fat (meat, cheese, etc.). Great for snacking, salad topping or for use in your favorite recipes.

Macadamia nuts are considered by many to be the world's most delicious nut. They're crunchy and creamy at once, with their own unique and delicious flavor. They are also a very nutritious, high-energy food, full of protein and fiber, and have the highest amount of beneficial monounsaturated fats of any known nut. Perfect for raw food recipes (creamy puddings, smooth veggie dips, divine nut patés) or for eating right out of the bag—just be sure to share!

Pecans are a good source of heart-healthy mono-unsaturated oils, easily-digested protein, vitamin E, folic acid, calcium, copper, magnesium, manganese, phosphorus, zinc and several B vitamins. Their sweet, buttery consistency makes them a fantastic snack or hiking food. Also great for making nut milks, nut patés, and healthy dessert recipes (they are a favorite for using in dehydrated cookie and pie "crust" recipes).

Pistachios are an excellent source of vitamin B-6, copper and manganese and a good source of protein, fiber, thiamin, and phosphorus. A recently published study reveals that pistachios pack in a variety of beneficial antioxidants and phytonutrients commonly found in tea (catechins), fruits, vegetables, red wine (anthocyanins) and soyfoods (isoflavones). The researchers conclude that pistachios are one of the best sources of antioxidants among plant-based foods. Pistachios are also one of the lowest calorie, lowest fat nuts. Pistachios have been shown to significantly reduce levels of low-density lipoprotein (LDL cholesterol) while increasing antioxidant levels.

Seeds

Hemp seeds, consisting of 33% highly digestible protein (containing 10 amino acids), are also rich in essential fatty acids, high in fiber, and contain chlorophyll, vitamin E, iron and trace minerals. Consisting of 35% oil, hemp seeds are packed with omega-6 and omega-3 and are the richest source of EFAs in the plant kingdom. These seeds have a delicious, nutty flavor that fits into almost any recipe. Sprinkle on your salads, add to salad dressings, smoothies, nut patés, homemade trail mixes and energy bars, etc. Made from hemp seeds, hemp protein powder is a whole food protein powder rich in complete protein (containing 50% protein) and beneficial branch chain amino acids. Add to your smoothies or shakes, or to your green juice drinks and green smoothies.

For centuries the Indians of the southwest and Mexico used the tiny chia seed as a staple food. Known as the "running food," its use as a high-energy endurance food has been recorded as far back as the ancient Aztecs. It was said the Aztec warriors subsisted on the chia seeds during the conquests. The Indians of the southwest would eat as little as a teaspoon full when going on a 24-hour forced march. Indians running from the Colorado River to the California coast to trade turquoise for seashells would bring only chia seeds for their nourishment.

Pumpkin seeds contain high amounts of trace minerals such as magnesium, manganese and phosphorus, which are important in brain health and development. Pumpkin seeds are also good sources of iron, copper, zinc and protein.

Sesame seeds are exceptionally rich in iron, magnesium, manganese, copper, and calcium, and contain vitamin B-1 (thiamine) and vitamin E (tocopherol). These seeds contain lignans, including sesamin, which are phytoestrogens with antioxidant

and anti-cancer properties. Sesame seeds also contain phytosterols associated with reduced levels of blood cholesterol. The
nutrients of sesame seeds are better absorbed if they are ground
or pulverized before consumption, as in tahini. Tahini, made
from husked (out-of-shell) sesame seeds, is a great component of
a healthy diet, and two tablespoons contain six grams of protein.
Tahini can liven up almost any kind of recipe. Use it to make
hummus (either traditional garbanzo bean hummus, sprouted garbanzo hummus, or even nut-based hummus—cashews work
great), rich, yummy salad dressings, sauces and dips, desserts,
etc.

Sunflower seeds are an excellent source of dietary fiber,
some amino acids (especially tryptophan), vitamin E, B vitamins
(especially vitamin B-1 or thiamine, vitamin B-5 or pantothenic
acid and folate), and minerals such as copper, manganese, potassium, magnesium, iron, phosphorus, selenium, calcium and zinc.
Additionally, they are rich in cholesterol-lowering phytosterols
and linoleic acid (an essential fatty acid).

Flax seeds are one of nature's best sources of two essential dietary components—Omega-3 fatty acids and lignan fiber.
They also contain an abundance of micronutrients. Flax seeds
may lower cholesterol levels, especially in women. Initial studies
suggest that flax seeds taken in the diet may benefit individuals
with certain types of breast and prostate cancers.

Poppy seeds are highly nutritious, and less allergenic than
many other seeds and nuts. Poppy seeds have been cultivated for
over 3000 years. Throughout history the plant has been revered
for its medicinal properties. In ancient Greece, poppy seeds were
introduced as medicine by Hippocrates. Sprinkle poppy seeds
over fruit or green salads, or add to creamy dressings. Poppy
seeds compliment sweet and savory food creations equally well.

Nutrition from the Sea and Lakes

Chlorella are microscopic plants that grow in fresh water. Chlorella gets its name from its chlorophyll content (highest of all known plants). Nutritionally dense, chlorella contains vitamins, minerals, trace minerals, essential fatty acids, chlorophyll and a vast array of phytonutrients. It is high in digestible protein. Many nutritionists and health advocates who have researched chlorella think it is one of nature's "perfect foods." Add to smoothies, green or vegetable juices and enjoy all the nutritional benefits chlorella has to offer.

Spirulina is a microscopic freshwater or saltwater plant. It is a whole-food, not a concentrate or extract. It is valued for detoxifying, as well as for its nutrient profile: high in vitamins, minerals, chlorophyll, antioxidants, and enzymes. Spirulina is a high-energy food. It contains all the B vitamins (which are themselves synonymous with high energy). It is alkalizing and helps keep the body from becoming overly acidic. Take powder or tablets with water, smoothies, or juices.

Thor's Hammer — As discussed in detail earlier in this book, Thor's Hammer is the perfect combination of two of the world's most powerful foods: chlorella and spirulina. Chlorella and spirulina are each considered by many in the health field as "perfect foods" — so it makes perfect sense to offer them together, in their purest form, in Thor's Hammer!

Aphanizomenon flos-aquae blue-green algae (AFA for short) is an all-organic, wild-harvested aqua-botanical that is considered by some renowned health authorities to be one of nature's most beneficial superfood. It can help restore overall body/mind balance by benefiting the immune, endocrine, nervous, gastro-intestinal and cardio-vascular systems. AFA provides 64 easily-absorbed vitamins, minerals and enzymes and biologically active chlorophyll. It is one of the most nutrient dense foods known. There are a few great AFA products I highly recommend: E3Live, Pure Klamath Crystals, Elixir of the Lake, Crystal Manna and Blue Manna.

Kelp, or "Wild Atlantic Kombu," (because of its similarity to Japanese Kombu) is "salty," yet low sodium, thanks to the rich complement of potassium, magnesium, and other mineral salts. Kelp is an especially rich source of potassium, iron, iodine, vitamin B-6, riboflavin, and dietary fiber. Kelp also contains a natural substance, glutamic acid, that enhances flavor and tenderizes. Phytochemicals in kelp have been shown to absorb and eliminate radioactive elements and heavy metal contaminants from our bodies.

An especially rich source of iron, potassium, iodine, vitamin B-6, riboflavin, and dietary fiber, dulse provides a complete array of minerals, trace elements, enzymes, and phytochemicals, as well as some high quality vegetable protein. It's a colorful salad ingredient, is tasty in raw soups, zesty with veggies, and boosts the flavor of any raw-food creation. Whole Leaf Dulse is soft and chewy, with a distinctive taste and a rich red color. It doesn't require any soaking, which makes it a great snack to be enjoyed right out of the bag.

Laver, also known as "Wild Atlantic Nori," is a purple/black, wild North Atlantic cousin to Nori—the seaweed processed into sheets for sushi (and raw vegan Nori Rolls!). Laver has a similar sweet and nutty flavor in an unprocessed form. This delicious, indigenous algae grows wild on the rocky shores of Maine from early spring to late fall. Of all the sea vegetables we carry at Rawpower.com, laver is the highest in Vitamins B-1, B-6, B-12, C and E. It also contains significant amounts of vegetable protein, fiber, iron and other minerals and trace elements. It isn't always easy to find nori sheets that aren't toasted. Raw <u>Nori Sheets</u> are great for making nori rolls with fresh vegetables, sprouts and nut patés, for making dehydrated treats, for snipping into salads, or for snacking on as-is.

<u>Alaria</u> is biologically and nutritionally very similar to Japanese wakame. In fact, it is so similar to its cousin of the Pacific, that it is referred to as "Wild Atlantic Wakame." Alaria, however, provides a more wild, yet delicate taste. Alaria's mild flavor profile allows it to blend in with many other ingredients without overwhelming them. It is the preferred sea vegetable for miso soup. Whole Leaf Alaria can also be marinated for use in salads, or dehydrated and enjoyed as "chips." Use in wakame salad recipes. Alaria is a good dietary source of vitamin A (beta carotene), iron, potassium, magnesium, chlorophyll, enzymes, trace elements, B vitamins and dietary fiber (contains more total dietary fiber—45%—and soluble fiber—16%—than oat bran).

Chondrus crispus, known under the common name <u>Irish moss</u>, or carrageen moss (Irish carraigĭn, "little rock"), is a species of red algae which grows abundantly along the rocky parts of the Atlantic coast of North America. In its fresh condition, the plant is soft and cartilaginous, varying in color from a greenish-yellow, through red, to a dark purple or purplish-brown. The principal constituent of Irish moss is a mucilaginous body, made of the polysaccharide carrageenan (contains about 55%). The plant also consists of nearly 10% protein and about 15% mineral matter, and is rich in iodine and sulfur. In the raw food community, Irish Moss is used in place of gelatin (an animal product) and other thickeners. When soaked, washed, then blended, Irish Moss disperses throughout the liquid it's in to create a semi-solid structure, much like "Jell-O!" Make raw ice-creams, parfaits, mousses, pies, meringues, etc.

<u>Sea Lettuce</u> is the "salad greens" of all sea vegetables. It is a deep-green sea vegetable with a distinctive flavor and aroma.

It is very high in iron and protein (similar to dulse), and is high in iodine and manganese as well. Like most sea vegetables, sea lettuce provides considerable amounts of dietary fiber (31%). Harvested and enjoyed worldwide, it is common in temperate and colder seas. Sea lettuce is good in raw soups or salads, but also delicious when eaten by itself. Experiment by tearing or cutting the whole dry leaves with scissors into your favorite dishes. Sea Lettuce is my favorite sea vegetable to munch on as-is!

Ocean's Alive Marine Phytoplankton is a unique micro-algae from the ocean and contains more than 90 ionic and trace minerals and is produced using a natural evaporation process employing the sun and the wind, which eliminates 93% of the sodium. Add a dropper-full of this Marine Phytoplankton to your smoothie or shake and experience this powerful superfood for yourself.

Fruits

Please note that, in this book, I'm using the botanical definition of fruit: a fruit is a food that contains the seeds within itself for regeneration of the plant. (Avocado, olive, tomato, cucumber, squash, pepper, etc. are all botanically fruits.)

Grapes are a form of berry. Like berries, grapes are highly nutritious with plenty of curative agents. They are great sources of vitamins A, B-1, B-2, B-6 and C, and also contain many health-promoting flavonoids. The deeper the color of the grapes, the richer the flavonoids. Grape phytochemicals such as resveratrol (a polyphenol antioxidant), have been positively linked to inhibiting cancer, heart disease, degenerative nerve disease, viral infections and mechanisms of Alzheimer's disease. Always strive to eat grapes containing seeds. Grape seeds are notable for their high content of tocopherols (vitamin E), phytosterols, and polyunsaturated fatty acids such as linoleic acid, oleic acid and alpha-linolenic acid.

Citrus fruits, such as oranges, grapefruits, lemons, limes, tangerines, etc., are also very important superfoods to the raw-foodist. They are very good sources of vitamin C and flavonoids. Oranges were historically used for their high content of vitamin C, which prevents scurvy. Scurvy is caused by a vitamin C deficiency, and can be prevented by having 10 milligrams of vitamin C a day. British sailors were given a ration of citrus fruits on long voyages to prevent the onset of scurvy, hence the British nickname of "Limey." Citrus fruits are notable for their fragrance, partly due to flavonoids and limonoids contained in the rind. The juice of citrus fruits contains a high quantity of citric acid giving them their characteristic sharp flavor. In the winter, citrus fruits are my number one choice of fruit.

Like berries, melons are another category of food that you should eat as many as you can get your hands on in the summertime. They're a good source of vitamin C and beta carotene and 90% plus water content—very hydrating. One thing to remember with melons is: eat them alone, or leave them alone—they do not digest well with any other foods.

One of my favorite foods, cherries, contain a red pigment called anthocyanins, which are potent antioxidants and deliver a variety of health benefits. Cherries have also been shown to help with inflammation and lower blood levels of cholesterol and triglycerides. Our family gets different varieties of cherries by the case from the farmers' market in the summertime.

Rich with heart-healthy oils and phytonutrients, raw olives make a great addition to any Mediterranean dish, are great on antipasto or tapas plates, and are perfect salad toppers—or just snack on them by themselves. Olives are the fruit richest in minerals such as calcium and magnesium and are the number one mucus dissolving fruit.

Most people are unaware of the fact that <u>avocados</u> have 60% more potassium than bananas. They are rich in B vitamins, as well as vitamin E and vitamin K. Avocados are also rich in fat—healthy fat, that is. In fact, about 75% of an avocado's calories come from fat. Fat from fruit sources is rare and should definitely be present in a raw-foodist's diet. Don't overdo it though—raw, fruit fat can still be fattening.

<u>Bananas</u> may not have the phytonutrient or antioxidant levels of other superfoods, but they are versatile and can serve multiple purposes in the diet of a raw-food bodybuilder. Bananas are also a natural antacid and can help keep your muscles from cramping. Bananas are approximately 95% carbs, 4% protein and 1% fat and contain moderate amounts of vitamin B-6, vitamin C, manganese and potassium. I use bananas as a carb "filler" for my post-workout smoothies and I also like bananas for their clean-burning caloric value. A medium-sized banana contains about 100 calories, so anytime I am a bit short on calories for the day, I'll eat a few bananas to get back to where I want to be. Bananas are an easy portable snack too.

<u>Lucuma powder</u> — This velvety, sweet fruit powder is the most popular dessert flavor in South America—outselling even vanilla and chocolate! Lucuma's rich aroma and full-bodied, maple-like flavor are perfect in everything from smoothies and raw cereals to home-made fruit "ice creams" and pies. Low-glycemic and an excellent source of fiber, beta-carotene, niacin and iron.

The <u>Mangosteen</u> is known as the "Queen of all Fruits." (Durian is known as the king.) Once only used in Traditional Chinese Medicine for its antioxidant, anti-inflammatory, antibacterial and antifungal qualities, mangosteen powder has achieved popularity with many interested in health. Put in smoothies for added antioxidant, vitamin and mineral value, as well as tangy, tropical flavor.

Others

Tocotrienols belong to the vitamin E family (tocopherals or tocols are the other group). Most of the vitamin E supplements available at local grocery and even health food stores are made using a cheap, synthetic version of alpha-tocopheral. Tocotrienols, on the other hand can be found in plant oils and cereal grains. Tocotrienol powder comes from raw, rice bran solubles. Because tocotrienol, like vitamin E, is fat soluble, avoid taking on an empty stomach. It is important to take this nutrient with fats (with nuts, seeds or oil in your smoothie, with a DHA supplement, etc.) and with or after other foods.

Jungle Peanuts — Actually a legume, these heirloom peanuts are quite possibly the ancestors of the commercial peanuts grown today. And the flavor? Subtle yet rich, aromatic and earthy. They're also a nutritional powerhouse—containing all eight essential aminos, plus methionine, with a whopping helping of the beautifying oleic acid. And they're loaded with protein, heart-healthy mono-unsaturated oil, vitamin E and much more. Unlike domestic peanuts, raw Jungle Peanuts are free of aflatoxin; plus, they're a sustainable rainforest product, harvested by indigenous peoples.

Mesquite Powder — If you know carob, you'll love its protein-rich cousin, mesquite! It has a complex, molasses-like flavor with a hint of caramel and blends well into smoothies. It adds thickness, sweet flavor and a smooth texture to many recipes. Used as a power food for centuries by the desert-dwellers of South America, mesquite contains calcium, magnesium, potassium, iron and zinc, and is also rich in the amino acid lysine.

Cacao (chocolate) has some beneficial properties (very high in antioxidants and magnesium) but can be a stimulant if too much is eaten, so be sure to use small amounts. I categorize cacao as a flavor, like vanilla or cinnamon. You wouldn't see someone making an entire meal out of vanilla or cinnamon, and the same thing goes for cacao. Many people enjoy adding cacao beans, nibs, powder or paste to smoothies for a raw "chocolate" smoothie or shake, or blending with raw sweeteners to make raw chocolate treats. Use cacao as a flavor, or as a once-in-a-while treat in a raw-food dessert.

There is evidence that aloe vera extracts are useful in the treatment of wound and burn healing, diabetes and elevated blood lipids in humans. These positive effects are thought to be due to the presence of compounds such as polysaccharides, mannans, anthraquinones, and lectins. Aloe vera juice is used for relief of digestive issues such as heartburn and irritable bowel syndrome.

Bee Pollen has been called "Nature's most nutritionally-balanced single Superfood." Packed with naturally occurring multivitamins, minerals, amino acids, enzymes and more, bee pollen is the pollen produced by flowers that honey bees gather and bring back to the hive. These pollen grains are microscopic in size, yet bees collect millions of these individual grains and bind them with nectar into small pellets. Beekeepers collect the pollen from the bees by placing a collection device at the entrance to the hive. This device gathers between 10% and 50% percent of the pollen that the bees are carrying, leaving plenty of pollen for the hive's needs.

Coconut oil is regarded by many to be the healthiest oil of all. It is mainly saturated fat, which is very different from the trans-fats everyone now knows we should avoid. Containing many protective nutritive factors, coconut oil included in the diet can give a boost to immune function. The best coconut oil comes from fresh coconuts that do not undergo a refining process but rather a centrifugal extraction process to derive the oil from the coconut. Coconut oil is perfect for many food preparation applications. Great for skin use, too! Use in place of moisturizers and lotions for skin healing and a vibrant glow.

*   *   *   *   *

For years, the pharmaceutical companies have been taking superfoods and extracting the medicinal qualities out of them—and making medicine to sell people at exorbitant prices. Now, everyone has access to these real, raw, superfoods. So, heed what Hippocrates (the father of Western medicine) once said: "Our food should be our medicine, and our medicine our food."

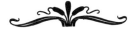

Thor's Raw Bodybuilding Menu Plan

People frequently ask me what I eat from the beginning of the day to the end. Well, it's always a little different, but there are some things that I highly recommend eating and drinking on a consistent basis: green-leafy vegetables, raw olives, celery, avocados, purple cabbage, coconuts, berries, bananas, distilled water, green juice, sea vegetables, Raw Power! Protein Superfood Blend, Thor's Hammer, and various raw superfood powders. Following is a sample menu plan that works great for me. Try it out and fine-tune it to fit your personal needs:

7:00am: 24-oz. distilled water (sometimes with lemon juice)

7:45am: Work out with weights (45 minutes, see Workouts chapter) Note: I am at my strongest and have the most energy when I have an empty stomach. No energy is being diverted toward digestion and more blood flow can be allocated to the muscles.

8:45am: Raw Power! Protein Smoothie and Thor's Hammer tablets (the most-important meal of the day). In a high-powered blender, add all of the following:

- 24-oz. fresh organic orange juice (or coconut water)
- 2-3 ripe organic bananas
- 1 cup frozen organic berries
- 2-3 scoops Raw Power! Protein Superfood Blend
- 1 teaspoon organic Acai Berry Powder
- 1 teaspoon organic Camu Camu Berry Powder

- 1 tablespoon Vitamineral Green
- 1 tablespoon Tocotrienols
- 120 Thor's Hammer tablets (taken with smoothie, not blended into smoothie, I take about 12-15 tablets per swig of smoothie)
(1050 calories, 52 grams protein, 8 grams fat)

10:15am: Two Raw Crunch Bars (Goji Berry or Blueberry) and 40 Thor's Hammer tablets
(340 calories, 17 grams protein, 20 grams fat)

11:45pm: Romaine lettuce salad with Raw Power Kalamata Olives (8-10), half an avocado, shredded purple cabbage, carrots, cucumbers, hemp seeds (1 teaspoon), homemade raw salad dressing and 40 Thor's Hammer tablets
(600 calories, 16 grams protein, 17 grams fat)

2:00pm: raw almonds, goji berries, goldenberries, romaine lettuce leaves and 40 Thor's Hammer tablets
(270 calories, 12 grams protein, 7 grams fat)

4:00pm: Cardio Workout (sports with my kids, hiking, running, swimming, Workout Swing, etc.)

5:00pm: 3-4 pieces of organic fruit and 20 Thor's Hammer tablets
(370 calories, 7 grams protein, 1 gram fat)

6:30pm: Romaine lettuce salad with Raw Power Kalamata Olives (8-10), half an avocado, shredded purple cabbage, carrots, cucumbers, hemp seeds (1 teaspoon), homemade raw salad dressing and 40 Thor's Hammer tablets
(600 calories, 16 grams protein, 17 grams fat)

8:00pm: 3-4 celery stalks and an apple
(140 calories, 3 grams protein, 0 grams fat)

9:00pm: Meditation and light stretching exercises

9:30pm: 12-oz. distilled water

Total for day: 3370 calories, 123 grams protein, 70 grams fat

I also take a few really good supplements (although not daily): Raw B-12, Vita Synergy multivitamin, and O-Mega-Zen (vegan Omega-3).

For those seeking a lower fat diet, simply decrease the amount of avocado, olives and Raw Crunch Bars. Those three foods comprise 52 of the 70 total grams of fat for the day. Also, 51 of the 123 total grams of protein come from Thor's Hammer tablets. Obviously I have built up to 300 Thor's Hammer tablets per day. This took me more than a year to build up to. I always recommend that people start with 20 tablets per day and build up slowly. The body needs time to adjust to this powerful superfood. (every 20 tablets = 3.5 grams of protein)

Try this menu plan (and variations of it) for 90 days. You should make substitutions to keep the diet interesting. For example, you can substitute zucchini for cucumbers, lettuce or cabbage wraps for salads, Maqui Berry powder for Camu Camu Berry powder, cashews, walnuts or pecans for almonds, Power Wraps for Raw Crunch Bars, etc. There are also some different smoothie recipes to choose from in the next section.

There are lots of ways to eat a raw-food diet. The Sample Raw Bodybuilding Meal Plan is specifically designed to fuel my body with enough calories and protein for maintaining and increasing muscle mass. Long distance or endurance athletes will need to eat more carbs (in the form of fruit) to avoid running their bodies at calorie deficits.

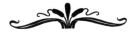

Raw Power
Workouts

*"A workout is 25 percent perspiration and 75 percent
determination. Stated another way, it is one part
physical exertion and three parts self-discipline.
A workout makes you better today than you were
yesterday. It strengthens the body, relaxes the mind
and toughens the spirit. When you work out regularly,
your problems diminish and your confidence grows.
A workout is a personal triumph over laziness and
procrastination. It's the badge of a winner—the mark
of an organized, goal-oriented person who has taken
charge of his or her destiny. A workout is a wise use
of time and an investment in excellence. It is a way
of preparing for life's challenges and proving to
yourself that you have what it takes to do what is
necessary. A workout is a key that helps unlock the
door to opportunity and success. Hidden within each
of us is an extraordinary force. Physical and mental
fitness are the triggers that can release it. A workout
is a form of rebirth. When you finish a good
workout, you don't simply feel better.
You feel better about yourself."*

— George Allen, former NFL football coach

Over the past 25 plus years, I have tried dozens of different weight-training routines. Some produced average results,

some produced good results, and one has produced excellent results. The routine which has produced excellent results is the one I have stayed with the last few years. And until now, I've never shared this routine with anyone.

This weekly routine consists of just three core weight-lifting exercises I do, each twice a week. They are very easy to remember, are very effective, and can be performed solo or with a training partner. Each lasts a little over 45 minutes, and each builds strength and endurance like nothing else I've ever found. Before I outline these three exercises in detail, first let me tell you what led me to them.

For many years, I overtrained—massively overtrained, in fact. Sylvester Stallone once said, "Overtraining wasted thousands of hours of my life." I can identify with that statement, although instead of the word "wasted," I'd say that overtraining used up thousands of hours of my life that could have been used to be productive in other areas of my life. Exercising is never "wasted time" to me, and I'm sure Stallone would ultimately agree.

So, for years and years, I overtrained until I got married and had four children (translation: very little time for myself anymore). After a few years of fatherhood, running a hectic business, and frequently missing workouts, I found myself needing to come up with some workouts which I could get the most out of, in the least amount of time. Obviously the Challenge at the Health Food Store (see Protein chapter) was a huge revelation, but how could I use that experience to help me with my time constraint challenge?

Over the next few years, one thing led to another and I finally nailed down three "perfect" workouts (at least for me). They consist of two different upper body workouts and one lower body workout. All three involve exercising core muscle groups, meaning you are using most of your main muscle groups (abdominals, back, chest, etc.), at the same time, and not isolating any particular body part. This helps on many levels, including developing good muscular symmetry and keeping everything "on the same page." For instance, you don't want to have strong abdominals, but a weak back, or any such similar problem. Not working out one's whole body equally and proportionally can lead to injury. This practice is like building a brick wall without mortar. Sooner or later, the wall is going to crumble.

Following is my weekly workout schedule, followed by the detailed routines:

Sunday: Hiking and/or sports with my kids, no weights
Monday: Upper Body 1
Tuesday: Upper Body 2
Wednesday: Lower Body
Thursday: Upper Body 1
Friday: Upper Body 2
Saturday: Lower Body

On all three workouts you'll need to use a timer and begin each set exactly every five minutes. Some people may read this and think that a set every five minutes is too much rest time. Believe me, by the time you get to sets six through ten, you won't think so.

I've found that using a timer keeps me on task and, when someone sees you using a timer, they are reluctant to disturb you while you're working out. I use a timer that goes off every five minutes—you can get them at a local store or on ebay for a couple of bucks.

Following are my exact workouts, including the weight

poundages that I currently use. Of course, this has taken me quite a while to build up to these poundages and you'll have to find the poundages that you can lift. Just start where you're at and don't worry about the poundages if they look meager to others. It's very important to complete all 30 reps per set. If you can't do 30 reps on all 10 sets, then decrease the poundage until you can.

On the 10th sets of both Upper Body workouts, I do as many reps as I can (30 plus)—this is my burnout set and I just keep going until muscular failure. Within 30 minutes after my workout, I drink my Raw Power protein/superfood/fruit smoothie with my Thor's Hammer tablets to help me refuel and replenish glycogen stores, provide high-quality protein and super nutrition to my muscles, and help speed up recovery.

*   *   *   *   *

Days: Monday and Thursday
Workout: Upper Body 1 (High-rep chest, arms and endurance)
Equipment: Two dumbbells, one flat padded bench

Take a dumbbell in each hand and lie down on a flat bench, with your feet on the floor for balance. Start with the dumbbells at each side of your chest, just below your pectoral muscles. Press them simultaneously upward until your arms are almost locked out, then lower them back to the starting position. That is one rep.

Set	Time	Weights	Reps
1	0:00	2 x 40s	30
2	5:00	2 x 50s	30
3	10:00	2 x 75s	30
4	15:00	2 x 100s	30
5	20:00	2 x 100s	30
6	25:00	2 x 100s	30
7	30:00	2 x 75s	30
8	35:00	2 x 75s	30
9	40:00	2 x 50s	30
10	45:00	2 x 50s	30+

The above may not look like a difficult upper body workout at first glance (or "difficult enough" to experienced weight trainers), but I'd bet the majority of current NFL football players couldn't do my Upper Body 1 45-minute workout with the poundages and repetitions I presently use, and I'm 42 this year, so I'm obviously doing something right! I have doubled my strength and endurance with this workout, while easily steering clear of injuries.

The next workout, Upper Body 2, was designed directly from my experience at the Health Food Store Challenge (as told back in the Protein chapter).

Days: Tuesday and Friday
Workout: Upper Body 2 (Challenge Exercises)
Equipment: Two dumbbells

Stand up straight and hold a dumbbell in each hand, hanging at arm's length. Next, curl both weights forward and up, holding your elbows steady at your sides and twisting your wrists slightly, bringing the thumbs down and little fingers up. Curl the weights up to the fronts of your shoulders, then twist them so your thumbs are closest to your head. Then press them up over your head to full extension. Bring them straight down to your shoulders and then back down to your sides again. That is one rep. Be sure to use dumbbells that you can do 30 reps with. This workout will be tough until you're used to it. For some people, 30 reps of even a light weight can be difficult. Unless you're an experienced weight-lifter, just start with light weights—like 5 or 10-pound dumbbells for women and 15 or 20-pound dumbbells for men.

Set	Time	Weights	Reps
1	0:00	2 x 40s	30
2	5:00	2 x 40s	30
3	10:00	2 x 40s	30
4	15:00	2 x 40s	30
5	20:00	2 x 40s	30
6	25:00	2 x 40s	30
7	30:00	2 x 40s	30
8	35:00	2 x 40s	30
9	40:00	2 x 40s	30
10	45:00	2 x 40s	30+

If I'm feeling particularly strong on a given day, I'll use two 50-pound dumbbells on 3-4 sets in the middle of the workout. So, keep in mind you can do the same (with a poundage you can do the full 30 reps on, of course). And, just to change things up once in a while, I'll do the first couple sets, then do a set of 100 reps (with 40-pound dumbbells). I'll count this "super" set as the equivalent of four sets, rest ten minutes, then complete the remainder of the workout as usual. Throwing the 100-rep set in there makes this workout extra exhausting, but very effective!

*   *   *   *   *

The third and final workout is the Lower Body workout. However, when you've finished this workout, it won't feel like you worked only your lower body!

Days: Wednesday and Saturday
Workout: Lower Body (High-rep Squats)
Equipment: One weight plate (or nothing!)

Stand straight up, flat-footed, and hold a weight plate (I use a 45-pounder) with both hands against your lower chest (or if you're not using a weight plate, arms crossed over your chest). Head up, back straight, feet 16-18 inches apart. Squat until upper thighs are parallel to floor. Return to starting position. Inhale down, exhale up. That is one rep.

For most people, a weight plate will not be necessary (this is called the Freehand Squat). This lower body workout is great even without the weight plate. I actually recommend starting without a weight plate, then optionally adding one in after you're used to the workout. Another option for the advanced weight-lifter is to do this workout with standard barbell squats—resting a barbell across the back of your shoulders. This way, one can add all the extra weight they want.

Set	Time	Weights	Reps
1	0:00	1 45-lb plate	30
2	5:00	1 45-lb plate	30
3	10:00	1 45-lb plate	30
4	15:00	1 45-lb plate	30
5	20:00	1 45-lb plate	30
6	25:00	1 45-lb plate	30
7	30:00	1 45-lb plate	30
8	35:00	1 45-lb plate	30
9	40:00	1 45-lb plate	30
10	45:00	1 45-lb plate	30

This lower body routine can be really gruelling if you're not used to it. However, when you do get used to it, you will look forward to this workout, perhaps even the most of the three workouts. It makes you feel great all over.

Legendary founder of Brazilian Jiu-Jitsu Helio Gracie, who lived to the age of 95, once said, "Sickness enters through the mouth, and age enters through your legs." I've always kept this quote in my head on Lower Body workout days.

Many times after one of these workouts, or randomly during the day, I'll do a hundred or so abdominal crunches to help keep my abs super strong.

*   *   *   *   *

So there you have it—my current weekly weight-training routine. The one that has produced the best results (by far) out of the many dozens of routines I've done since I first started training with weights in junior high school.

I do this routine pretty much all year around, with brief breaks to "surprise" my muscles. It's wise to surprise your muscles periodically with different exercises or you may plateau, get bored, or your training and progress may suffer. I like to surprise my muscles with out-of-the-ordinary exercises like doing shoulder press reps with full 5-gallon water bottles—and since I live on an acreage in a northern mountain forest, it seems like I'm always moving and lifting trees and other heavy objects.

To greatly improve your balance, try lifting weights standing up on one foot at a time. Experiment! You'll find that your form and lifting mechanics sharpen up dramatically.

If you're an athlete training for a specific sport, then

you're obviously going to need to train a bit differently, according to your sport's needs. But for the person seeking to build super strength and build a massive, healthy, muscular physique, I think you're going to love these three routines.

Jack LaLanne once said, "Going one day without exercising is like committing suicide." Now, I wouldn't take that too literally, but Jack did have a point. The Law of Inertia states that a body in motion tends to stay in motion, and a body in rest tends to stay in rest. Even on my days off from weight training, I like to stay active. I've mentioned I enjoy playing sports with my kids: we play baseball, football and basketball, and we always take something to throw whenever we go to a park or beach. I also get a good workout coaching their sports teams. Other exercises I enjoy are: manual labor, running stairs, swimming, hiking and Workout Swing exercises.

A Workout Swing allows you to stretch, strengthen and tone muscles in ways which can be difficult to achieve at the gym or even at a yoga class. Made of high-quality parachute fabric, the Workout Swing is unique in that it offers you the ability to stretch and strengthen, but is also a therapeutic piece of equipment that can be used to practice inversion therapy (or inversion yoga) which is ideal for gentle, passive stretching and traction of the spine. Hanging upside down can alleviate muscular tension and pain as well as promote increased joint mobility and flexibility, increased relaxation and circulation of the blood, lymph and energy. All of these in turn promote good health and well being. The Swing is also extremely portable. It is lightweight, weighing under three pounds, and can easily fit into a backpack. Take it wherever you go and hang it from a tree or exposed beams. It also converts to a full size hammock for camping trips. The Swing appeals to anyone who is into any form of exercise or for those who just want to have fun. The material is comfortable enough against the skin and it breathes too, so you will never have that sweaty feeling. And the system is simple and quick to adjust from one level to another. Remember to start slow! Don't do too much, too soon. Most people haven't been upside down in years, and it will feel strange at first. Once you see how easy it is and how great it feels, you'll look forward to it. My kids wish they each had their own Swing, but we all share and take turns. To see one of my sons demonstrate a few exercises on the Workout Swing (exercises "even a kid can do!"), go to www.rawpower.com and type "workout swing" in the search box. You'll find the video on the page for the Workout Swing.

                *   *   *   *   *

Note: The original printing of my Raw Power! book contained long, intense workouts with several different exercises and a more comprehensive Definition of Terms. I no longer train with these workouts, or even recommend them, but I'll put them online and if you'd like to check them out, send me an e-mail and ask me for the online link to the routines.

                                        — thor@rawpower.com

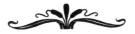

Definition of Terms and Proper Execution of Raw Power Exercises

<u>Abdominal Crunches</u>: Lie on your back on the floor. With your knees bent, raise your legs and place your feet against a wall or bench for support. Place your fingertips on your temples. Raise your head and shoulders toward your knees with a sit-up motion and simultaneously lift the pelvis and feel the contraction of the abdominals as the upper and lower body crunch together. Flex the abdominals to get the fullest possible contraction.

<u>Aerobic Exercise</u>: With oxygen. The muscles' demand for oxygen is met by the circulation of oxygen in the blood. Examples are: walking, swimming, long-distance running, bicycling, etc.

<u>Anaerobic Exercise</u>: Without oxygen. The oxygen demands of the muscles are so high that the circulatory system cannot supply adequate oxygen. Examples are: weight-lifting, sprinting, wrestling, etc.

<u>Barbell</u>: A long bar with weights at both ends, designed to be used by both hands at once.

<u>Cardiovascular Training (aka Cardio)</u>: Cardiovascular training is an integral part of overall conditioning. These exercises strengthen the heart, lungs, and circulatory system. See *Aerobic Exercise*.

Challenge Exercises: Stand up straight and hold a dumbbell in each hand, hanging at arm's length. Next, curl both weights forward and up, holding your elbows steady at your sides and twisting your wrists slightly, bringing the thumbs down and little fingers up. Curl the weights up to the fronts of your shoulders, then twist them so your thumbs are closest to your head. Then press them up over your head to full extension. Bring them straight down to your shoulders and then back down to your sides again.

Dumbbell: A short bar with weights at both ends, intended for use with one hand at a time.

Dumbbell Bench Presses: Take a dumbbell in each hand and lie down on a flat bench, with your feet on the floor for balance. Start with the dumbbells at each side of your chest, just below your pectoral muscles. Press them simultaneously upward until your arms are almost locked out, then lower them back to the starting position.

Repetition (rep): One complete exercise movement, from starting position, through the full range of movement, then back to the beginning.

Set: A group of repetitions (reps). The number is arbitrary. Programs designed to produce cardiovascular fitness generally use high-repetition sets, while those that aim for strength use fewer repetitions.

Squats (barbell): With the barbell on a rack, step under it so that it rests across the back of your shoulders, hold on to the bar to balance it, raise up to lift it off the rack, and step away. Keeping your head up and your back straight, bend your knees and lower yourself until your thighs are just lower than parallel to the floor. From this point, push yourself back up to the starting position.

<u>Squats (freehand)</u>: Stand straight up, flat-footed, arms crossed over your chest. Head up, back straight, feet 16-18 inches apart. Squat until upper thighs are parallel to floor. Return to starting position. Inhale down, exhale up.

<u>Squats (with weight plate)</u>: Stand straight up, flat-footed, and hold a weight plate (I use a 45-pounder) with both hands against your lower chest (or if you're not using a weight plate, arms crossed over your chest). Head up, back straight, feet 16-18 inches apart. Squat until upper thighs are parallel to floor. Return to starting position. Inhale down, exhale up.

<u>Superset</u>: A set of two or more exercises performed in a row without stopping (zero rest).

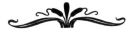

Recipes for Strength and Muscle Building

This chapter includes some simple raw-food recipes I have found to help build strength and muscle over the years. All of the recipes are easy to make and can be adjusted to suit your taste and needs.

Raw Power Protein Smoothies, Shakes and Fresh Juices

Raw Power! Protein Superfood is designed to be blended or added into your homemade shakes and smoothies. Always strive to use fresh, raw, organic ingredients — your body will thank you for it!

Another thing I think is really important is to invest in a high-quality blender, which virtually liquifies food for a quick meal and optimal absorption. I use the Vita-Prep commercial blender with variable speed knob. I've had one for almost 15 years, and my wife, kids and I use it every day. (We sell them at Rawpower.com for only slightly above our cost. It's a great deal and I guarantee you it will be your most-used kitchen appliance!)

Basic Raw Power Smoothie

2 scoops Raw Power! Protein Superfood Blend (any flavor)
2 cups (16 oz.) fresh organic orange juice (or other fresh juice), fresh coconut water or fresh nut milk

Blend a Basic Raw Power Smoothie with any of the following ingredients of your choice to make your own delicious super smoothie:

* fresh fruits: bananas, peaches, mangoes, etc.
* fresh or frozen berries
* leafy greens
* green powders (Vitamineral Green, Pure Synergy, etc.)
* berry and fruit powders (Fruits of the Earth, acai powder, goji berry extract, camu camu powder, mangosteen powder, etc.)
* dates (pitted)
* agave syrup
* chlorella powder
* spirulina powder
* etc.
* For super nutrition, take Thor's Hammer tablets with your daily smoothie.

<u>Thor's Ultimate Superfood Meal</u>

2 scoops Raw Power! Protein Superfood (Green)
1 tablespoon Fruits of the Earth blend
24 ounces fresh organic orange juice (or pure water)
1 ripe organic banana
1 cup of frozen organic berries (strawberries, blackberries, raspberries, blueberries, etc.)
1 handful organic raw/organic goji berries
1 tablespoon raw/organic acai berry powder
1 teaspoon raw/wildcrafted camu camu berry powder
1 teaspoon raw/wildcrafted mangosteen powder

Blend all ingredients until desired consistency. Then,

depending on your tablet-swallowing capabilities, with each swig of your smoothie, take 3-15 Thor's Hammer tablets.

This super meal contains approximately 40 grams of protein and little to no fat, and has countless health benefits. Massive nutrition...truly one of the healthiest meals anyone is eating!

Basic Raw Power "Shake"

2 scoops Raw Power! Protein Superfood Blend (any flavor)
2 cups (16 oz.) fresh organic orange juice, fresh coconut water or fresh nut milk

Shake in a container with lid. Because they don't require a blender, these shakes are easy and you can make them anywhere: on the go, at the office, etc.

Bazler Kids' Favorite Smoothie (serves 4 or 5)

4 cups fresh orange juice and/or fresh nut milk (usually a combination of both)
1/2 cup Raw Power! Protein (Vanilla)
2-3 tablespoons green powder, (examples: Vitamineral Green, Pure Synergy, Greener Grasses, Perfect Food, etc.)
3 pitted dates
1 frozen banana (optional)
2 cups frozen fruit (peaches, apricots, nectarines, berries, cranberries—we freeze them when they're ripe)

Hint from Jolie: even just a bit of dark berries like blueberries, blackberries, and huckleberries will mask the color of the greens and give the smoothie a nice color (greenish/brownish smoothies can sometimes be a turn-off to the young or skeptical!).

Choco/Vanilla Raw Power Smoothie

Blend:
1 scoop Raw Power! Protein (Chocolate)
1 scoop Raw Power! Protein (Vanilla)
1 ripe banana
2 cups (16 oz.) of fresh coconut water or nut milk
pitted dates or agave syrup to adjust sweetness

Creamsicle Raw Power Smoothie

Blend:
2 scoops Raw Power! (Vanilla) Protein Superfood Blend
8 oz. fresh organic orange juice
8 oz. fresh nut milk
sweeten to taste with dates or agave syrup

Super Green Raw Power Smoothie or Shake

Blend:
2 scoops Raw Power! Green
2 cups (16 oz.) fresh organic celery/cucumber juice or other green veg juice

Amanda's Banana Almond Milkshake

1/2 cup raw almond milk
1-2 bananas (depending on size)

Recipes for Strength and Muscle Building   133

2 tablespoons flax, hemp or other good omega oil
2 scoops Raw Power Protein (Original)

Blend all ingredients for a few seconds. Add ice and blend, adding more ice until it reaches milkshake consistency. This is usually sweet enough without sweetener, but you can always add agave syrup for those with a serious sweet tooth!

Amanda's "Frawppuccino"

1 cup raw almond milk
2 tablespoons raw carob (or mesquite) powder
1 tablespoon (roughly) of raw cacao powder or nibs
Agave syrup to taste (maybe a couple of tablespoons - you may add more if you are really needing the sugar rush!)
1 scoop Vanilla Raw Power Protein
1scoop Chocolate Raw Power Protein (or just double up on the Vanilla)

Blend ingredients together with enough ice to give it the "Starbuck's Frappuccino" consistency and enjoy! Always double blend to get a really great texture to the drinks. Once you add the ice, this makes a really large amount so prepare to share! Note: for those who are limiting their cacao intake, you can always omit the cacao and add a bit more carob or mesquite if needed.

Amanda's Vanilla Milkshake

1 cup almond milk
2 scoops Raw Power! Protein (Vanilla)
Agave syrup to taste (a couple of tablespoons for most people)

Blend ingredients with ice until it reaches "milkshake" consistency. This is a big hit with kids and a great summer treat!

Basic Green Juice

5 handfuls kale or other green (spinach, chard,
   dandelion greens, collards, etc.)
1 cucumber
3 stalks celery

Put all foods through juicer and enjoy.

Power Green Juice

3 handfuls one kind of green
3 handfuls another kind of green
1 cucumber
3 stalks celery
2 handfuls parsley
1-2 tablespoons Vitamineral Green superfood

Put greens, cucumber, celery and parsley through juicer. Stir in Vitamineral Green.

Captain's Powerhouse

1 young coconut
1 large avocado
2 handfuls wild or organic greens

Drain coconut water into Vita-Mix or blender. Crack coconut in half, scoop out the soft meat and add to Vita-Mix.

Scoop avocado with spoon and add to Vita-Mix. Add two hand-fuls of greens. Blend until smooth. (Drink 30 minutes after workout for best results.)

Purple Cabbage Juice

1 head purple cabbage

Put chunks of purple cabbage through juicer and enjoy. Juice the whole head of cabbage and drink immediately to receive all the medicinal benefits. This is a great once-a-month post-workout drink. As stated previously, purple cabbage is high in glutamine, an amino acid that plays an important role in protein synthesis, muscle growth and nitrogen donation for many ana-bolic processes.

Go-Through-a-Brick-Wall Juice

6 ounces sprouted wheatberries
6 handfuls of wild or organic dandelion greens
1 ounce ginger root

Put 3-day sprouted wheatberries through juicer. (For infor-mation on how to sprout wheat, read "The Wheatgrass Book" by Ann Wigmore.) Put ginger through juicer. Put greens through juicer. Pour juice into large glass. This drink is electrical—quite a jolt!

Fire Water

1 orange or red habanero pepper
1 medium orange

4 cups distilled water

Put habanero pepper in juicer. Peel orange and compost or discard orange peel. Put orange fruit through juicer. Pour 4 cups of distilled water into juicer to flush out remaining nutrients. Pour Fire Water into pitcher and serve. It is best to drink this 30 minutes before a meal.

<u>Datenut Shake</u>

1 cup soaked almonds (or other nut of your choice)
4-6 dates
distilled water

Remove and discard date pits. Blend soaked almonds and date fruits with distilled water to desired consistency.

<u>Post Running or Hiking Drink</u>

3 stalks celery
2 medium apples

Put foods through juicer. Excellent sodium/potassium balance.

Soups, Salads, Wraps and Snacks

<u>Avo Soup</u>

2 large avocados
1 medium cucumber
1 medium tomato
1/2 cup loose fresh corn

1 cup chopped zucchini
1/4 cup chopped green onion
1 tablespoon fresh cilantro
distilled water

Discard avocado pits and skins. Put 1-1/2 avocado, cucumber, tomato, and cilantro into blender. Blend, adding distilled water for desired consistency. Pour into a bowl. Chop remaining 1/2 avocado into small cubes and stir into soup, along with the zucchini, corn, and onions.

Daily Green Salad

Here is the green salad I eat almost every day, year-round:

4 cups chopped romaine lettuce
1/2 cup shredded or chopped purple cabbage
1 carrot, chopped
1/2 cucumber, chopped or sliced (if in season)
half an avocado, cubed or sliced
8-10 Raw Power Kalamata Olives
1 teaspoon hemp seeds

Toss all of the above then cover with your favorite homemade raw salad dressing.

Daily Vegetable Plates

My wife puts out a raw/organic vegetable plate for our family every day (or brings one with us when we're on the go). These include: broccoli, cauliflower, purple cabbage (cut in large chunks for grabbing and crunching), celery, carrots, fennel, cucumbers, zucchini, kohlrabi—whatever is in season. If you make a container full of washed and simply-cut vegetables and take it with you, you'll have veggies for snacks at work, on-the-go, or whatever you may be doing. Vegetable plates aren't just for parties!

Avocado Salad

3-4 handfuls wild or organic greens
2 large avocados
10-20 Raw Power Kalamata Olives
1 tablespoon extra-virgin cold-pressed olive oil
1 medium orange

Discard pits of olives, pits and skins of avocados, and orange peel. Make a bed of wild or organic greens and/or herbs, add avocado, olives, olive oil, and add juice of the orange to taste. Greens and healthy, raw fats are body builders. A powerful salad!

Applenut Salad

1 head romaine lettuce
1 cup sunflower sprouts
1 diced apple
1/2 cup chopped walnuts
1 cup grapes

Make a bed of lettuce and sprouts. Put apple, walnuts, and grapes on top of bed.

Raw Power Cabbage Wraps

2 large avocados
1 handful diced green onion
1 handful chopped cilantro
1-2 red (ripe) jalapeno peppers, seeded and diced (optional)
1 medium tomato
1 head purple cabbage
1 yellow (ripe) lime

 Mix ingredients avocados (skins and pits removed), onion and jalapeno peppers. This is your wrap filler. Spoon out filler into unbroken purple cabbage leaves (or you can use raw, organic nori sheets or romaine lettuce leaves), squeeze lime juice onto filler, and wrap each leaf around filler to create these delicious and satisfying wraps.

Ants in a Canoe

2 large apples
2 cups soaked almonds
2 ounces raisins (with seeds if possible)

 Soak almonds in distilled water for 12 hours. Put soaked almonds through a Champion or Green Power Juicer, using the blank plate. This will make an almond paste (or you can use already-prepared raw, organic almond butter). Cut apples into quarters. Remove and discard seeds. Spread almond butter on apples then cover with raisins. Great snack.

Thor's Ultimate Raw Trail Mix

1/2 cup almonds
1/2 cup walnuts
1/2 cup pecans
1/2 cup cashews
1/2 cup Hunza raisins
1/2 cup dried goji berries
1/2 cup dried, whole-leaf seaweed (laver or dulse)

Mix all together in a bag (powerful combo!).

           *   *   *   *   *

Note: Agave syrup (also known as agave nectar) is a raw, vegan substitute for sugar and honey. Smoother, sweeter, and lower on the Glycemic Index, it's a favorite of those who prefer sustainable energy vs. the post-sugar blues. Organic blue agave syrup is made exclusively from the finest blue agave plants. This syrup is perfect for raw dessert recipes, smoothies, teas, and many more delicious creations.

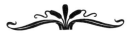

Questions and Answers
with Thor

Over the years I've been asked *a lot* of questions pertaining to the raw-food diet and lifestyle. In this section, I've listed some of the most frequently-asked questions and my answers.

*   *   *   *   *

Q: What is the main reason to adopt a raw-food diet?

A: Because you want to, because you enjoy it. I can't stress this enough. I have seen so many people adopt a raw-foods lifestyle for the wrong reasons, and these people invariably fail and actually hinder their personal advancement and potential. I've seen people do it because "it's healthy," and they agonize over eating their salad greens while what they really want to be eating is a plate of rice, beans, fish (or whatever). Yet they keep choking down the raw foods because "it's healthy." They are ingesting a lot of bad energy and cannot be truly happy or liberated, or healthy for that matter, even though that's their outward reason for doing it. I've seen people do it because it seems elitist. These are the type that look down on anyone who is "not enlightened" and make others feel uncomfortable rather than sharing wanted information. These people usually lose a lot of friends and alienate their families. They also cannot be truly happy or liberated. There is nothing elitist about the raw-food diet, it is just a diet and lifestyle choice. And I've seen people do it to fit into the associated raw social scene. Again, the main reason, the ONLY reason, to adopt a raw-food diet is because you want to, because you enjoy it.

*   *   *   *   *

Q: What have been the most positive health benefits raw-food-ism has brought to you? What do other raw-foodists say?

A: Feeling vibrant and alive is the benefit that first comes to mind for most raw-foodists, myself included. A feeling of well-being and healthfulness. Living with more clarity and consciousness. Improved senses are another benefit: improved eyesight, sense of smell, hearing, a clean taste palate, increased touch sensation. A heightened sixth sense, intuition, is also part of that.

*   *   *   *   *

Q: What exactly is a raw-food diet, how do you define raw-foodism, and what does someone have to do, in practice, to be a raw-foodist?

A: It is simply the natural way to nourish your body. A raw-foodist is not something one becomes; a raw-foodist is something that all living creatures on Earth already are. We are designed to eat raw foods. Food in its raw, natural state cannot be nutritionally improved upon, especially not by cooking it. Raw-foodists take all their nourishment from raw, natural foods—unadulterated by cooking.

*   *   *   *   *

Q: So, what's wrong with cooked foods?

A: Because cooked food is part and parcel to civilization, we have been trained never to question it. Perhaps some of the first widely-eaten and shared cooked food started as cooked mash that accompanied the vegetables, fruits, nuts and seeds people were eating. And perhaps humans adapted to that pretty well, especially over time. But now, in present-day society, what constitutes the basis of human nourishment is canned and boxed food coming out of the roaring jaws of huge industrial factories, and the flesh and milk of animals being churned out by factory farms. (Not to mention the chemicals and other dangerous non-food stuffs put in our foods and used to grow our foods.) Shelf-life and transportability are all-important in our food industries, and the benefits of fresh foods don't matter to most of those who sell us our food. There are now many, many people who actually eat a 100% cooked diet, never eating any fresh fruits or vegetables at all (which is crazy!) and the incidence of disease and human illness has never been higher. The fact that we as a culture haven't really questioned cooked food has resulted in us being completely out of balance in our dietary and food-growing practices, as a whole and as individuals. The basis of human nourishment is clear to me: it is RAW PLANT FOOD, which is presented to us in abundance in nature.

*   *   *   *   *

Q: At what point does a person see results or notice a difference? After years of raw-foodism? Months? Days?

A: It's definitely not an overnight transformation, although you can start to see results immediately. You wouldn't expect to be in perfect physical shape by working out once. And the same is true with anything, for that matter. Fundamentals practiced daily and consistently produce the desired results. For me, all these years later, it's still a journey I'm experiencing and enjoying every day.

Q: What other lifestyle changes do you espouse besides adopting a raw-food diet?

A: Eating only organic and wild foods. The commercial food of civilization is unfit for consumption and transforms people into mutants. Yes, that's harsh, but reality is harsh. Pesticides and genetically-modified foods are not acceptable for the true health-seeker. Humanity cannot improve upon natural foods with poisons and laboratory experiments.

*   *   *   *   *

Q: Have you changed other areas of your life as radically?

A: The change to raw foods was not that radical. Raw foods are our natural foods. Captain Crunch cereal is radical; cotton candy is radical; hot dogs are radical. Raw plant foods are common sense.

*   *   *   *   *

Q: What are some more factors in overall health besides diet?

A: Along with nutrition, people must make certain the other requirements of the body are met. These include: cleanliness, exercise, rest, clean air, deep breathing, adequate sunshine on the skin, stretching, massage (being touched by others), intelligent thinking, loving relationships, interaction with animals, and abstinence from artificial indoor heating and cooling as much as possible. I mention cleanliness first because I feel that a lot of people that get into raw foods start to move away from civilized living—and that's great, to a point. It's important to untangle oneself from the mess of contemporary culture, but when one scoffs at personal hygiene and cleanliness because it's "not natural" or "cooked" to bathe, it's not healthy for them or the raw-food movement in general. It really boils my blood when I see someone that is supposed to be setting an example, trying to be a "picture of health," but they stink of body odor and have nasty, dirty hair, fingernails and skin. The skin is the largest eliminative organ of the body. Toxins and impurities are pushed to the surface of the skin and need to be washed off. I can tell you right now that if you are living or working anywhere near automobiles, factories, cities, roads, highways, or neighborhoods, you need to be bathing every day. Your outside appearance is a reflection of your internal health. One cannot be truly healthy if one is filthy. (In addition, always use a shower filter. You either filter out what is coming onto and into your body, or you *become* a filter.)

$$*\qquad*\qquad*\qquad*\qquad*$$

Q: Have you ever encountered hostility from others when you discuss raw foods?

A: Sure, but mostly I've encountered positivity and open ears. Some people have a hard time when their belief systems are challenged. Because talking about raw foods is part of my business, my work, I seldom talk about it in my personal life. I see people get into trouble when that's all they ever talk about, or they cram it down people's throats, or they make others feel uncomfortable around them because they are so judgmental. Anyone like that is a bore. As with anything, what you have to say about raw foods will fall on deaf ears unless the recipient is truly interested and unless they have initiated the conversation. I don't try to convince anyone of anything, but share information when it's wanted.

$$*\qquad*\qquad*\qquad*\qquad*$$

Q: What do you eat when you go to a restaurant or go to someone's house for dinner?

A: Almost every restaurant serves a salad, and some are even pretty good. When you go to someone's house for dinner and you do not think there will be much or anything for you to eat there, offer to bring a fruit or vegetable salad, or fruit or vegetable plate.

*   *   *   *   *

Q: Do you carry your own food everywhere?

A: When I travel, yes, I take some food with me. Airplane food is definitely not an option! I have traveled all over the world and have never had any trouble finding good food. Sometimes I hear people complain about not having raw, organic food in their area; chances are they're simply not looking hard enough. I always bring Raw Power! Protein, Thor's Hammer and a few other essential items wherever I go.

*   *   *   *   *

Q: Is wheatgrass really a natural thing for humans to eat? Don't you have to grind it up in a machine to make its nutritional value accessible?

A: While wheatgrass may not the most natural food for us, I believe in its healing and cleansing properties and I think it is a vital part of the transition and detoxification process. (See Ann Wigmore's Wheatgrass Book for more information.)

*   *   *   *   *

Q: Do you think it's relevant to have a scientific basis to promote your idea?

A: "Science" is a tricky thing because you can prove almost anything with scientific studies, yet there will always be contradictory information from other scientific studies. That is why I am more inclined to use common sense and instinct. There have been a lot of recent studies showing the benefits of raw-foods, and I think as time goes by, raw-foodism will be normalized the way vegetarianism and veganism are now.

                *   *   *   *   *

Q: What do you think of medicine, or better, of doctors as professionals in health?
.

A: Medical doctors are coming around and some are even beginning to support a raw-food diet. There is obviously a place in our modern society for doctors and western medicine. (I went to a doctor/hospital when I was in a serious car accident and would go for any kind of life-threatening emergency like that.) But the way the medical community is set up right now is disappointing: doctors having very little education on nutrition and holistic practices, patients not taking responsibility for their own health, an over-prescribing of pharmaceutical drugs, etc.

                *   *   *   *   *

Q: What do you think of drugs and medicines? Why do so many people use them?

A: Drugs and medicines are toxic substances, and I think there are few cases where their benefits outweigh their ill effects. People use them because they are looking for a "magic pill" instead of taking their health into their own hands, and because drugs and medicines are over-prescribed by doctors and heavily pushed by the pharmaceutical giants. Most people don't know any better, and just blindly follow their doctor's orders, and most doctors are trained to treat illnesses and pathologies with drugs.

Q: Do you take any nutritional supplements?

A: Yes, I take superfoods and raw supplements now. At first, I was totally into the 100% raw purist thing, then I learned more about really high-quality superfoods and supplements, and I'm glad I did. One can develop deficiencies even on a vegan raw-food diet. All the really successful, super-healthy, long-term raw-foodists I know eat a balanced raw-food diet consisting of organic, mineral-dense fruits, vegetables, nuts, seeds, superfoods, and raw supplements.

* * * * *

Q: Are raw beans or grains part of a raw-foodist's diet?

A: Beans and grains can be difficult to eat raw and they are not so pleasing to the taste palate for many people. They can also be hard on the digestive system for some. There are many other choices for those who don't do well with raw, sprouted beans and grains. For protein, green-leafy vegetables, Raw Power! Protein Blend and Thor's Hammer are good choices. Filling and grounding foods include avocados, olives, coconuts, durians, seeds, and nuts. The raw-foodists who do use sprouted beans and grains usually add small amounts of sprouted beans to big green salads or nut or seed loaves, and add sprouted grains to dehydrated, raw granolas or seed crackers or that sort of thing. The key is using these in smaller amounts. Over-indulging in raw beans or grains can result in an awful stomachache!

* * * * *

Q: You say that, "food-combining principles were formulated by and for cooked-food eaters, they don't pertain to you." This sounds very much like some statements in T.C. Fry's Healthful Living Newsletter of many years ago, saying that food-combining was for the biologically compromised (sick) and not always necessary for persons of robust health. Since many of the recipes in your book combine fruits, nuts, and vegetables in a blender and so forth, might you elaborate upon this for the readers?

A: Food combining rules are for people with poor absorption and poor digestion and are not always necessary for healthy people. My cycles change and my diet changes, I eat varying combinations now, and that's what makes me feel great. The combinations that work for me may not necessarily work for others, and vice versa.

* * * * *

Q: What sort of detoxification effects does the average person experience when they start adopting a raw-food diet?

A: It really depends on how you lived your life before. Someone who abused his or her body with deleterious substances is obviously going to have a heavier detoxification than someone who lived more healthfully. When the body buried in unprocessed residues of cooked food and/or other substances finally has the energy to release them, it will.

* * * * *

Q: I notice that you advocate colon irrigations. To many natural hygienists it was a blessing to be free of such dogma to simply allow their bodies to heal through "intelligently doing nothing." Why direct your readers to this non-hygienic Dr. Ehret-esque "mucusless" mentality?

A: In some cases, there are residues in the body (gall stones, impacted fecal matter, etc.) that are "stuck." As with the amalgam fillings people want removed from their mouths, intestinal residue removal may have to be assisted mechanically. Colon irrigation isn't necessary for everyone, but decades of eating fragmented, clogging foods can't always be eliminated by the body through proper eating.

$$*\qquad*\qquad*\qquad*\qquad*$$

Q: Can a raw foodist overdose on a particular food or eat too much of one food?

A: Yes, definitely. One should learn how to keep oneself balanced on raw foods. A balanced raw-food diet consists of the three essentials: greens, sugars, and fats. These foods balance against each other and keep you centered. It's different for everyone. Someone may be able to eat only cherries for days when they first come in season, and they may feel great. While another person couldn't eat only cherries for half a day without feeling unbalanced. Each person needs to find their own balance.

$$*\qquad*\qquad*\qquad*\qquad*$$

Q: On a raw foods diet you are putting a very high quality "fuel" into your system. It seems as though it is easy to spend a lot of money quickly eating a totally raw organic diet. Any advice for someone having trouble dishing out the extra cash?

A: I keep the costs low by eating what is in season. Obviously, eating something like cherries in the winter is going to be expensive because cherry harvest season is summer (plus, those cherries at the market in winter are probably from the other side of the planet, which is another problem as far as sustainability goes). Also, eating what is in season is nature's way of telling you what to eat. (Note: For these reasons, I included the Seasonal Produce Availability section in this book which lists the peak seasons for all fruits and vegetables.) Another thing to consider is to never penny-pinch when it comes to your health. You can penny-pinch somewhere else in your budget, but definitely not on your health and diet. People who aren't willing to pay for the highest-quality foods now are going to get less than excellent results in their health and vitality—and those results could end up with visits to a doctor or hospital, which will be much more expensive than organic produce.

Another tip: We knew a single working mom who needed to feed her kids healthfully while keeping to her modest family food budget. While the mother was away at work, her kids (who were older) were allowed three "free" foods that they could have whenever they wanted and as much as they wanted: carrots, cabbage and apples. All three of these foods are affordable and easy to come by in large quantities (huge bags of carrots, bags or boxes of apples, and cabbage heads bought 2-3 heads at a time).

*   *   *   *   *

Q: A lot of people's first reaction to a raw-food diet is "I could never do that..." or "I just couldn't give up..." What would you say to these people?

A: I'd say, "Yes, you will be giving up many lifeless, poisoned foods that are unhealthy and doing your body and soul an extreme disservice. You will be stepping outside your comfort zone and experiencing something totally new and amazing. You will experience for the first time in a long time (or maybe in your life!) feelings of well-being, vibrancy, and euphoria far better than any drug high. Your new-found taste buds will wake up from their numbness and experience hundreds of new fresh, high-quality, delicious foods. You will meet some amazing people on your journey—people who are not a part of the herd; people who are part of the solution, not part of the problem; people with insights, stories, and lessons. You will look back on your old life and see that your comfort zone was never comfortable at all."

*   *   *   *   *

Q: Is a raw-food diet for everyone?

A: No. A raw-food diet is for people with a success-consciousness—a strong desire to better themselves physically, mentally, and spiritually. The raw-food diet is for people who wish to advance toward their full potential. It's a shame that the vast majority of people on this planet have little or no concern for these things.

*   *   *   *   *

Q: Your Raw Power Program is said to be the only program about building strength and muscles naturally (raw). What is the general idea behind it?

A: My program is about how to have the body that you've always desired—a fit, strong, healthy, and vibrant body. Many people now know that a raw-food diet is the natural way to eat, but some people have difficulty building strength and gaining healthy muscular weight on raw foods. The Raw Power Program is about overcoming those difficulties and attaining a high level of health, eating a 100% natural diet (all raw or very high raw), true natural bodybuilding, and total fitness. The only way to build your body naturally is through eating naturally.

*   *   *   *   *

Q: What is your concept of bodybuilding, and how does it differ from similar activities, such as weight training for conditioning, powerlifting, and Olympic-style weightlifting?

A: My concept of bodybuilding is building and maintaining a super-strong and super-healthy body, free from illness and disease. My program combines natural bodybuilding, weight-lifting, total fitness, conditioning, and diet information that is specifically designed for building and maintaining muscle and strength.

*   *   *   *   *

Q: Does your program appeal to bodybuilders only?

A: Actually, competitive bodybuilders probably make up a small portion of those who follow the Raw Power Program. My program appeals to anyone with a desire to better themselves mentally and physically. Just as many women as men have read past editions of this book and found the information applicable and helpful. The same can be said about the book/program appealing to just as many non-athletes as athletes. Raw Power appeals to everybody, whether you want to look like a raw version of Arnold Schwarzenegger, or you just want a slim, muscular body capable of increased energy and stamina.

*   *   *   *   *

Q: Do you recommend maximum lifts? Why or why not?

A: I don't do maximum lifts anymore. This is because I prefer to train alone and also because I'm really into high reps now. It's obviously not wise to do maximum lifts without a training partner or spot. Training alone has its downfalls for some people, but, at this point in my life, I cannot tolerate a gym atmosphere (smells, air conditioning, terrible music, crowded, etc.). Another interesting thing to note is that when I used to go to the gym, as soon as someone found out that I didn't eat cooked food, meat, pills, or steroids, I would become an attraction. People would watch me work out, which I hate. I would end up talking about the raw-food diet and my workouts would suffer. If you have a quality training partner and are in great shape, I see no reason why you couldn't perform maximum lifts.

*   *   *   *   *

Q: What do you think your potential would be if you did conventional bodybuilding?

A: The potential of anyone eating unnaturally is a short term gain at the expense of a long term tragedy. Sure, you can build huge muscles eating meat all day and injecting steroids and guzzling pills and commercial protein powders, but there is a tremendous price to pay in the end.

*   *   *   *   *

Q: For all-raw training, what is the difference for someone who has already experienced conventional bodybuilding versus someone who has no prior bodybuilding experience? Who usually has better success?

A: It's really an individual thing. The people that make building strength and muscle naturally their number one priority are always going to find more success than the people that want something for nothing. I love observing and meeting people that are my peers as far as dedication and motivation; it pushes me closer to my full potential. A person can either have "champion mentality" or "spectator mentality," the choice is theirs.

*   *   *   *   *

Q: What are your current "vital statistics." Besides your height and weight, would you also reveal your blood pressure, and heart rate, as well as the girth measurements of your neck, shoulders, chest, arms, forearms, wrist, waist, hips, thighs, calves, and ankles?

A: I'm currently 6'2" and 245 pounds, and my blood pressure at my last physical was 110 over 72. I'm not really into all that girth measurement stuff; the only measurements that matter for me are how strong I am and how vibrant I feel. I used to measure my arms when I was younger, but I realize now that measurements prove very little. Though its arms aren't very big, a chimpanzee can rip a car door off of its hinges. I've seen "bodybuilders" with 22-inch arms that can't benchpress 300 pounds. I'm going for chimpanzee strength, not big measurements.

                    *   *   *   *   *

Q: What are your reasons for bodybuilding? Is it because you are vain and ego-centric, as some critics accuse bodybuilders of being? I mean, why do it? Why not just relax and stay skinny? Since lot of people think that bodybuilding is a waste of time and energy, what would you say to convince someone that they should body build?

A: I like feeling strong, and I like the feeling of being pumped up. I don't try to convince anyone of anything. I'm just presenting information showing that one can gain weight and muscle on a raw-food diet and without undermining one's health with unnatural nutrition.

                    *   *   *   *   *

Q: Don't you have a reason beyond feeling strong and pumped as motivation to lift weights?

A: Arnold Schwarzenegger once said that being pumped up

feels better than an orgasm! I don't know if I would go that far, but he has a good point! Being pumped up feels great, and I have yet to be in a bad mood after a good workout. That's my motivation for lifting weights, to feel great.

*   *   *   *   *

Q: Why do some raw-food eaters seem to be lacking the "definition" and "vascularity" that most cooked food bodybuilders have?

A: I have long thought that definition is not always healthy (concentration camp prisoners all had definition!). In my opinion, the massive, defined, ripped, professional bodybuilders of today have accepted the ultimate Faustian bargain. They fill their bodies with absurd nutritional pollution just to look "defined." Then they wonder why they have completely broken down (or died) by the time they are "middle-aged." Muscle definition has a lot to do with genetics and body type. My brother and I have worked out with weights just about every day for the last 25 years (I'm talking hard-core workouts), and we are very strong, but we're not the most "ripped" guys in the world. I don't worry about it. Nature determines your natural body type. Think of your health first and foremost, the definition will either be there or not. The race for the lowest body-fat percentage is a kamikaze crash-course.

*   *   *   *   *

Q: Many animals do show vascularity and muscle striations in their natural state. Mightn't we also? I used to think definition was genetic, too, until I was all raw and finally saw all of my abdominal muscles in clear awesome cuts. Might not diet be the deciding factor on definition and vascularity?

A: Well, I have found that my definition was "best" when I was in my twenties, when I was eating a more conventional body-builder-type diet. But since I've been into raw foods, I'm much stronger and I feel much better. That's all I really care about. If I can't see all my abdominal muscles in clear awesome cuts, I don't care as long as I feel great. And you're correct, many animals do show vascularity and muscle striations in their natural state, and many animals do not, yet they are very strong and powerful. (Hippos are some of the most berserk, muscular, strong creatures on the planet, and they have almost no "definition.")

*   *   *   *   *

Q: Where do you get enough protein for real muscle growth?

A: Where does a cow, rhinoceros, hippopotamus, or gorilla get enough protein for real muscle development and growth? Raw plant foods. Protein synthesis is protein synthesis.

*   *   *   *   *

Q: I have heard it takes about a year to build ten pounds of muscle tissue. Do you feel that the ten to fifteen pound range is about the maximum growth curve that a raw body builder has?

A: I don't ever put limitations on anything. If someone wanted to gain, say, 20 pounds of muscle in a year, it could be done. It fully depends on the conviction, persistence, and determination of the individual.

*   *   *   *   *

Q: Would you explain why coconut and avocado are necessary for you and whether there may be another way to gain weight if one doesn't want to, or can't, go the coconut and avocado route?

A: Fat is the delivery device to the muscles and bones of minerals drawn from green-leafed vegetables. One could use olives, nuts, seeds and/or their oils (olive oil, hemp oil, etc.) instead of coconuts and avocados. I personally enjoy all of them. (Olives are one of the best foods for bodybuilding.)

*   *   *   *   *

Q: How can one gain more weight on one or two large meals, as you recommend, rather than on many small meals throughout the day?

A: This slows down the metabolism, allowing one to more easily gain weight. It is very simple and demonstrable to anyone who tries it. Keep in mind that almost every helpful weight loss program has one doing just the *opposite*: eating small frequent meals throughout the day to speed up metabolism.

*   *   *   *   *

Q: You mention fasting once a month, yet some would say that it is unnecessary or even harmful to fast this often if one is already eating a biologically correct diet. Would you explain the reasoning behind your fasts?

A: Again, this slows the metabolism. The digestive organs need an occasional rest. The whole body does. Every animal in nature has times of fasting or leaner food supplies, and humans used to also. But in our modern living systems, most of us have regular access to food year-round throughout our lives, so the body doesn't get that metabolic break. (One should only fast if it feels right.)

*   *   *   *   *

Q: How often do you work out with weights?

A: Six times a week for a little over 45 minutes each workout. I used to work out for a lot longer, but since I have many obligations now—a family, a homestead, and a fast-growing business—I had to come up with shorter, more effective workouts (see Workouts chapter).

*   *   *   *   *

Q: Do you find that the raw-food diet tends to make high-rep training more the way to go rather than high-poundage training?

A: Combining the two would be optimal. High-reps with high-poundage!

*   *   *   *   *

Q: You stated that one should train in the sun whenever possible. This is a refreshing change from the solar phobia of skin cancer warnings that we hear these days. What are the benefits of training in the sun?

A: Increased blood flow in the muscles, increase testosterone levels, fresher air, and the opening up of stagnated, contracted areas of the body.

*   *   *   *   *

Q: Do you ever take layoffs?

A: Yes, when I go on trips. It is good to give your body a rest once in a while so when you come back, you are fresh and motivated.

Q: You mention that sexual abstinence is desirable to help conserve body nutrients before exercise or competition. Isn't this just an old wives' tale perpetuated by trainers to keep their athletes away form the distraction of a new romance?

A: No, it definitely is a reality. If one is constantly draining one's sexual energy, it makes strength gains more difficult. Two closely-matched training partners that have the difference of one being sexually active and one not will notice the strength/stamina difference. This is not to imply complete sexual abstinence, but abstinence before workouts and competitions.

*   *   *   *   *

Q: You use free weights, right? Why do you prefer them?

A: Free weights allow for a free range of motion, and they require the individual to use her/his own balance. I have found that when I concentrate on mechanics (form), I get a much better workout.

*   *   *   *   *

Q: Do you use any aerobics in your training?

A: Yes, I enjoy hiking, swimming, running stairs, family bike rides, and Workout Swing exercises. I also play a lot of sports with my kids: baseball, basketball, football, wrestling, sparring and grappling (my kids train in martial arts), you name it.

*   *   *   *   *

Q: What should a very young all raw bodybuilder know regarding his special considerations?

A: Start where you are. Build up slowly. Don't try to do everything at once.

*   *   *   *   *

Q: Is your program useful to the advanced bodybuilder?

A: Definitely. Before now, I doubt the advanced bodybuilder has come across information that says one can be super-strong without wearing one's body down prematurely with unnatural, artificial substances and cooked foods.

*   *   *   *   *

Q: How much time do you think someone should devote to taking care of his/her body?

A: The goal is to make healthful choices every waking hour of the day. In our culture, we often take better care of our material possessions than our bodies, and taking care of one's body is often seen as vain. My wife has this quote: "If you don't take care of your body, where will you live?"

*   *   *   *   *

Q: Do you think we have any "duty" to live as Nature intended, or is it just something we can do if we personally value Nature?

A: I feel it is our moral and ethical obligation to live consciously and conscientiously. What we eat deeply and radically affects how we think, feel, and behave, it directly affects how we interact with the planet. In that sense, it is a duty. Switching to a raw-food or high-raw diet has many positive implications for the environment, as well as ourselves.

Q: What do you see as the biggest challenge a raw foodist must deal with in everyday life?

A: Dealing with the rules, regulations, traditions, customs, and red tape of a dead society. It drives me crazy! People think they are free but they are not. Try walking down the street the way you came into the world (nude) and see what happens, see if you're really free. Eating raw foods at least liberates you and allows you to step outside of the current global consciousness and see what is really going on.

*   *   *   *   *

Q: Is there a philosophy, spirituality, or ethics behind raw-foodism, or is it just about health benefits?

A: Raw-foodism impacts every aspect of your life: mental, emotional, spiritual, and physical. So while health benefits may be what prompts a person to raw-foodism, once they adhere to it, they begin seeing the ecological and ethical impact and realizing and appreciating the spiritual benefits.

*   *   *   *   *

Q: Tell us about your raw food company.

A: Rawpower.com is an internet and mail order business and we also supply health food stores with raw, organic foods, super-foods and supplements. Our mission statement reads as follows: "We believe in eating as locally, seasonally, and sustainably as possible. We also believe there are many worthwhile additions to local and seasonal eating, like nuts and seeds, dried fruits and berries, raw-food snacks, natural oils, whole food supplements (as opposed to synthetic), etc. We've made it our business to carry and distribute these worthwhile "additions," as well as helpful kitchen and household items and healthy lifestyle products and resources. We take great care in choosing our products because we care about you, our customers."

We offer products to support individuals and families in enjoying a healthy, and thus vibrantly fuller, life. In addition to foods, we offer books, CDs and DVDs, juicers, dehydrators, water filters, sprouters, and many more raw lifestyle products. We sell the items we use in our own lives, items we know other people want to buy and use too. Our catalog and inventory grow larger all the time as we add more select products.

We feel strongly about putting a lot back into the raw-food community. We have spent years networking, meeting other raw-foodists around the world, reviewing and adding new products to our catalog, and connecting people in order to make the raw-food community successful and welcoming to new-comers.

*   *   *   *   *

Additional questions can
be emailed to Thor at:
thor@rawpower.com

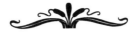

Seasonal Produce Availability

The seasonal availability of fruits and vegetables is Nature's way of telling you what to eat and when. Eating foods when they are in season is an integral part of health and the importance of doing so cannot be overemphasized. Thus, I have included the following information regarding seasonal produce availability. Though varieties of each food may differ by region, this compilation lists each food's peak season/availability according to a survey of Farmers' Markets conducted within the United States. (All Seasons = foods that are generally available year-round. "Best" in chart = best selection of food type can typically be found at that time of year.)

Food	Season
Acorn Squash	Late Summer, Fall
Almond	Fall
Ambrosia Melon	Summer
Apple	Fall, Early Winter
Apricot	Summer
Arame	All seasons
Artichoke	Fall
Arugula	Year-round/best in colder months
Asian Pear	Fall, Early Winter
Asparagus	Spring
Atemoya	Late Winter, Spring
Avocado	All seasons
Banana	All seasons
Basil	All seasons
Beet	All seasons

Food	Season
Blackberry	Early Summer
Black Sapote	Summer
Blood Orange	Winter
Blueberry	Summer
Bok Choy	Winter, Spring, Summer
Boysenberry	Early Summer
Brazil Nut	Fall
Breadfruit	Early Summer
Broccoli	Year-round/best in colder months
Brussels Sprouts	Late Fall, Early Winter
Cabbage	Winter, Spring, Summer
Canistel	Spring
Cantaloupe	Summer
Carambola	Spring
Carob	Spring
Carrot	All seasons
Casaba Melon	Summer
Cashew Apple	Fall
Cassia	Spring
Cauliflower	Year-round/best in Fall, Winter
Celery	Year-round/best Summer, Fall
Chard	Year-round/best Spring to Fall
Chayote	Fall, Winter
Cherimoya	Late Winter, Spring
Cherry	Early Summer
Chestnut	Fall
Chicory	Fall, Winter, Spring
Chive	All seasons
Cilantro	All seasons
Cranberry	Fall
Crenshaw Melon	Summer
Coconut	All seasons
Collard	Year-round/ best in colder months
Corn	Summer

Food	Season
Currant	Spring
Cucumber	Summer
Dandelion	Late Winter, Spring
Date	Fall, Winter
Dill	All seasons
Dulse	All seasons
Durian	Spring, Summer
Eggplant	Summer, Fall
Endive	Fall
Escarole	Fall, Winter, Spring
Fennel (bulb fennel)	Winter, Spring, Summer
Feijoa	Fall
Fiddlehead Fern	Summer
Fig	Summer
Frisee	Fall, Winter, Spring
Garlic	All Seasons
Ginger	All seasons
Ginseng	All seasons
Goji Berry	Summer
Gooseberry	Summer
Gourd	Fall
Grapefruit	Winter, Early Spring
Grape	Summer
Green Bean	Early Summer
Green Butter Lettuce	Fall, Winter, Spring
Green Leaf Lettuce	Fall, Winter, Spring
Green Oak	Fall, Winter, Spring
Guava	Spring
Hazelnut	Fall
Hijiki	All seasons
Honeydew Melon	Summer
Huckleberry	Summer
Jakfruit	Spring
Jicama	All seasons

Food	Season
Jujube	Fall
Kale	Year-round/ best in colder months
Kiwi	Winter, Early Spring
Kohlrabi	Year-round/abundant in Summer
Kombu	All seasons
Kumquat	Winter, Early Spring
Lamb's Quarters	Late Winter, Early Spring (wild)
Leeks	Year-round/abundant Fall - Spring
Lemonberry	Summer
Lemongrass	Winter
Lemon	Winter, Early Spring
Lime	Winter, Early Spring
Loganberry	Early Summer
Longan	Summer
Loquat	Early Summer
Lotus	All seasons (imported)
Lovage	Spring, Summer
Lychee	Summer
Macadamia Nut	Fall
Mache	Year-round/greenhouse grown
Malva	Late Fall, Winter
Mamey Sapote	Spring
Mango	Late Spring, Summer
Mangosteen	Fall, Early Summer
Marjoram	All seasons
Mint	All seasons
Mizuna	Year-round erratic availability
Monstera Deliciosia	Late Spring, Summer
Mountain Apple	Spring
Mulberry	Summer
Mustard Greens	Early Winter to Sprin peak
Nasturtium	Summer
Nectarine	Summer
Nori	All seasons

Food	Season
Okra	Summer
Olive	Fall, Winter, Spring
Onion	All seasons
Orange	Winter, Early Spring
Oregano	All seasons
Papaya	All seasons
Parsley	All seasons
Parsnip	Late Fall to Early Spring
Passionfruit	Fall
Peach	Summer
Peanut	All seasons
Pear	Fall, Early Winter
Pea	Spring
Pecan	Fall
Pepper	Late Summer, Fall
Peppergrass	All seasons
Persimmon	Fall
Pineapple	All seasons
Pine Nut	Fall
Pistachio	Fall
Plantain	All seasons
Plum	Early Summer
Pomegranate	Fall
Pomelo	Winter
Potato	Year-round/best in Summer, Fall
Prickly Pear	Fall
Pumpkin	Fall
Purslane	Summer
Quince	Fall, Early Winter
Radicchio	Fall, Winter, Spring
Radish	Year-round/peak in colder months
Rambutan	Summer
Raspberry	Early Summer
Red Butter Lettuce	Fall, Winter, Spring

Food	Season
Red Oak	Fall, Winter, Spring
Red Orach	Fall, Winter, Spring
Rhubarb	Spring (never eat rhubard leaves!)
Rosemary	All seasons
Rutabaga	Late Fall
Sage	All seasons
Sapodilla	Spring
Savory	Fall, Winter, Spring
Scallion	All seasons
Sea Palm	All seasons
Shallot	All seasons
Sharlyn Melon	Summer
Snow Pea	Early Spring to Early Summer
Sorrel	Early summer to Fall
Sourgrass	All seasons
Soursop	Late Winter, Spring
Spinach	Winter
Strawberry	Early Summer
Sugar Apple	Late Winter, Spring
Summer Squash	Spring to Summer
Sunchoke	Fall, winter
Sunflower	Late Summer
Surinam Cherry	Spring
Sweet Potato	Available Late Fall to Spring
Tamarind	Spring
Tangelo	Winter, Early Spring
Tangerine	Winter, Early Spring
Tango	Fall, Winter, Spring
Tarragon	All seasons
Tat Soi	Fall, Winter, Spring
Thyme	All seasons
Tiger Lily	Summer
Tomatillo	Late Summer
Tomato	Summer

Food	Season
Travissio	Fall, Winter, Spring
Turnip	Winter
Ugli Fruit	Winter, Early Spring
Velvet Apple	·Late Summer
Violet	Summer
Wakame	All seasons
Walnut	Fall
Watercress	Fall, Winter, Spring
Watermelon	Summer
Wheatgrass	All seasons
White Sapote	Winter, Summer
Wintercress	All seasons
Winter Squash	Fall, Winter
Yam	Fall
Zucchini	Early Summer

Again, this list is an estimate for seasonal produce availability. Availability can vary greatly from region to region. The best guage for what is seasonal where you live is what is available at your local and regional farmers' markets.

*   *   *   *   *

Nuts have been stored by humans and other creatures since the beginning of nuts! While nut crops have seasons, they store well in cool places so they are readily available year-round.

*   *   *   *   *

There thousands more edible foods in the world (over 50,000!). You could eat a different raw plant food every day of your life and *still* not try them all! Does anyone still think eating a raw-food diet is boring?

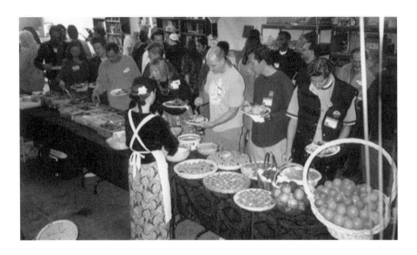

A spectacular array of raw gourmet dishes served at one of our raw-food events. Jolie's food is amazing!

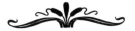

Conclusions

To go places you have not gone,
you have to do things you have not done.

As mentioned at the beginning of this book, once one knows of and experiences a raw-food diet first hand, one can never think about food and diet the same way again. It is eye-opening, there's no doubt about it. For most health seekers, finding the perfect diet is a never-ending journey, not a destination. Even after all these years of doing raw foods, I am constantly learning new things and discovering more "pieces of the puzzle." In closing, here are some last words of inspiration and food for thought:

* Maintain your emotional poise. Release worry, fear, anxiety, jealousy, stress, nervousness, and neurosis through physical movement of the body—through the free flow of body energy, and through deep breathing. Take your aggressions out by engaging in anaerobic exercise.

* Be true. The only fools are those who fool themselves. The idea that natural nutrition can be followed by unnatural and harmful effects is an absurd notion which should be abandoned once and for all.

* Nutrition is no science—it is very simple. Live by the laws of nature and you shall prosper; live by the laws of civilization and you shall suffer.

 * All weight loss and emaciation due to a raw-food diet is a result of the "good pushing out the bad" and other catabolic detoxification processes. The strength and weight will build if one is persistent.

 * A major problem plaguing humanity is addiction. Addiction to toxicity; addiction to being in a toxic physiological condition, actually. People are constantly trying to reach a level of euphoria artificially—a euphoria which is already theirs naturally.

*   *   *   *   *

When you are 100% raw for an extended period of time, it is a life-transforming experience. Again, there is no magic pill, but there is a magic process to achieving vibrant health. Try it for yourself...and you'll be convinced.

How many of these things do you do on a daily basis?:

 * get outdoors in fresh air and the sun and experience nature
 * exercise vigorously
 * associate with positive people
 * think powerful thoughts
 * delve into the mysteries of life
 * drink freshly-made protein/superfood smoothies and juices
 * eat huge, creative salads
 * avoid mass media, television and other time- and
       mind-wasters
 * live in a place that is conducive to good health (fresh, clean
       air, low crime rate, local recreational opportunities, etc.)
 * have (or find) a really cool, balanced partner to share life
       with

Your life is either a chore or a celebration.
The choice is yours.

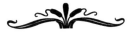

Contact Us

If you have any questions or comments about any of the material contained in this book, feel free to contact Thor or the Raw Power Staff.

To receive free monthly e-mail newsletters (concerning new products, monthly specials, exciting news, media coverage, etc.) from Thor and Raw Power, sign up quick and easy at:

www.rawpower.com

or send an e-mail to:

thor@rawpower.com

Additional copies of Raw Power! may be ordered directly from Rawpower.com or by calling Raw Power Customer Service. Bulk book discounts and many health-related products are also available.

Thor Bazler
Raw Power
PO Box 1358
Coeur d'Alene, ID 83816 U.S.A.
(208) 676-9065
1-877-846-7708 toll-free customer service

Internet:
www.rawpower.com

Thor's Main Raw Power Bodybuilding Products

Book: Raw Power!...$14.95
Raw Power Protein Superfood Blend (Original)...........$29.95
Raw Power Protein Superfood Blend (Chocolate)..........$29.95
Raw Power Protein Superfood Blend (Green)................$29.95
Raw Power Protein Superfood Blend (Vanilla)..............$29.95
Raw Power Protein Superfood Variety 4-Pack...............$95.84
Thor's Hammer pressed tablets (1000 count)...............$34.95
Goji Berries, Raw Power brand (raw, organic)..............$12.95
Hemp Protein Powder, Raw Power brand (raw, organic)..$16.95
Vitamineral Green, superfood powder (500g / 17.6 oz)...$59.95
Kalamata Olives, Raw Power brand (raw, unsprayed)......$12.95
Vita-Prep Commercial Super Blender..........................$449.95

These, and many more awesome products, are on sale online at
Rawpower.com. All prices are subject to change.

All Raw Power brand products are Raw, Certified Organic
and/or Wildcrafted: the highest quality products on the market.

Quantity discounts are available for all Raw Power products.

For an extensive listing of **Raw Power products**,
please visit our state-of-the-art,
online Raw Organic Superstore at:

www.rawpower.com

Or call us at 1-877-846-7708.

Raw, organic foods, supplements, books,
21st century kitchen appliances
and much more...